THE BIOMECHANICS OF AMATEUR BOXERS

by

SARAH STOJSIH

THESIS

Submitted to the Graduate School

of Wayne State University

Detroit, Michigan

in partial fulfillment of requirements

for the degree of

MASTER OF SCIENCE

2010

MAJOR BIOMEDICAL ENGINEERING

_____
Advisor   Date

_____

_____

UMI Number: 1481056

All rights reserved

INFORMATION TO ALL USERS
The quality of this reproduction is dependent upon the quality of the copy submitted.

In the unlikely event that the author did not send a complete manuscript
and there are missing pages, these will be noted. Also, if material had to be removed,
a note will indicate the deletion.

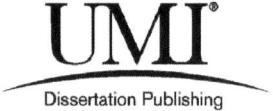
Dissertation Publishing

UMI 1481056
Copyright 2010 by ProQuest LLC.
All rights reserved. This edition of the work is protected against
unauthorized copying under Title 17, United States Code.

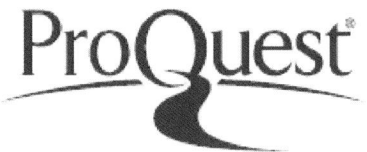

ProQuest LLC
789 East Eisenhower Parkway
P.O. Box 1346
Ann Arbor, MI 48106-1346

ACKNOWLEDGEMENTS

The National Operating Committee on Standards for Athletic Equipment, United States Amateur Boxing Association, and Wayne State University provided funding for this research project. In addition to funding provide, the author would like to acknowledge partial support from the Anthony and Joyce Danielski Kales Scholarship. The author would like to thank her advisor, Dr. Cynthia Bir, and her committee members, Dr. Albert King, and Dr. Marilyn Boitano for all of their guidance, support, and expertise.

Impact Boxing Headgear was developed for this study by Simbex, Inc. and the IBH data was post-processed by Jonathan Beckwith of Simbex, Inc. Dr. Kenneth Podell assisted in the post-processing of the neurocognitive data. I would like to acknowledge all the athletes who took time from their busy training schedules to participate in our study. Special thanks are extended to Don Sherman, Nate Dau, and Hai-Chun Chien for assisting in data collection and analysis. In addition, a special thanks to Dr. Marianne Wilhelm, Erin Hanlon, Charlene Brain, Richard Bolander, Osmar Pinto Neto, and Jacob Mack for assisting in data collection. I would also like to thank the leadership of the Safety/Equipment Committee and supporting Staff of the United States Amateur Boxing Association for their commitment to safety and Ringside for allowing data collection during their annual tournament.

TABLE OF CONTENTS

Acknowledgements ii

List of Tables v

List of Figures vii

CHAPTER 1- INTRODUCTION 1

    1.1 Problem Statement 1

    1.2 Background and Significance 1

    1.3 Specific Aims 7

CHAPTER 2 - BRAIN INJURY 9

    2.1 Types of Brain Injuries 9

    2.2 Head Injury Mechanism and Injury Prediction 13

    2.3 Diagnostic Tools 16

CHAPTER 3 19

    3.1 Introduction 19

    3.2 Methodology 21

    3.3 Statistics 25

    3.4 Results 26

    3.5 Discussion 31

CHAPTER 4 – BIOMECHANICS OF SPARRING 39

    4.1 Introduction 39

4.2 Methods 41

4.3 Statistical Analysis 51

4.4 Results 52

4.5 Discussion 59

CHAPTER 5 – BIOMECHANICS OF COMPETITION 64

5.1 Introduction 64

5.2 Methods 65

5.3 Statistical Analysis 68

5.4 Results 68

5.5 Discussion 74

CHAPTER 6 – CONCLUSIONS AND FUTURE RECOMMENDATIONS 79

6.1 Conclusions 79

6.2 Future Recommendations 82

APPENDIX A – HIC Approvals 84

APPENDIX B - A Prospective Study of Punch Biomechanics and Cognitive Function for Amateur Boxers 88

APPENDIX C – Standardized Assessment of Concussion (SAC) Forms A and B 94

References 96

Abstract 106

Autobiographical Statement 108

LIST OF TABLES

Table 3 1 Descriptive characteristics of sample population   22

Table 3 2 Mean punch force and hand velocity for each punch type by gender   27

Table 3 3 Mean head acceleration and injury criterion for each punch by gender 29

Table 3 4 Correlations between punch dynamics and risk of injury parameters for female athletes   30

Table 3 5 Correlations between punch dynamics and risk of injury parameters for male athletes generated by the jab punch   31

Table 3 6 Comparison of biomechanical data found in literature   32

Table 3 7 Mean biomechanical data classification by weight class   36

Table 4 1 Descriptive statistics for mean IBH impact data   52

Table 4 2 Descriptive statistics for peak IBH impact data   52

Table 4 3 Correlation between weight and risk of injury parameters for male athletes   53

Table 4 4 Correlation between weight and risk of injury parameters for female athletes   54

Table 4 5 General locations and corresponding mean accelerations and injury severity   57

Table 4 6 Mean ImPACT scores for baseline, post, and 24 hours post bout tests   58

Table 4 7 Comparison of data found in literature for male boxers   60

Table 5 1 Mean and peak IBH impact data   69

Table 5 2 General locations and corresponding mean accelerations and injury severity   72

Table 5.3: Mean sub-scores and overall SAC scores......................................73

Table 5.4: Cognitive scores and peak head acceleration comparison......................74

Table 5.5: Differences between SAC scores at baseline and immediately following bout..77

LIST OF FIGURES

Figure 3.1: Example of head acceleration data collected from HIII............................28

Figure 3.2: Translational headform accelerations produced by female and male athletes..33

Figure 3.3: Rotational headform accelerations produced by female and male athletes.34

Figure 3.4: HIC values produced by female and male athletes.................................34

Figure 4.1: Instrumented Boxing Headgear...44

Figure 4.2: IBH system recording data..44

Figure 4.3: Linear regression of IBH acceleration data and HIII 3-2-2-2 acceleration data..46

Figure 4.4: General impact locations 47

Figure 4.5: Male and female translational accelerations for each impact...................54

Figure 4.6: Male and female rotational accelerations for each impact.......................55

Figure 4.7: Male and female HIC scores for each impact..55

Figure 4.8: General locations for each impact sustained...56

Figure 4.9: Rotational and translational accelerations of each impact based on general location...58

Figure 5.1: Translational head accelerations for each impact....................................70

Figure 5.2: Rotational head accelerations for each impact..70

Figure 5.3: HIC scores for each impact...71

Figure 5.4: General locations for each impact sustained...72

Figure 5.5: Overall baseline and post-bout SAC scores..73

CHAPTER 1- INTRODUCTION

1.1 Problem Statement

The main objective in amateur boxing is to land the highest number of clean punches to the opponents head or torso. Although the goal is to outscore an opponent, the surest way to victory is with a knockout. Consequently boxers strive to land blows to the head. During amateur boxing bouts, the athletes are required to wear protective headgear and heavily padded gloves to aid in energy absorption (Dau et al., 2006). Even though precautions are implemented acute and chronic head injuries are still a problem. A study found that approximately half of the injuries that occur during an amateur boxing competition are concussions (Porter and O'Brien, 1996).

While injuries produced from participation in boxing are known, the mechanics behind what causes the injuries have been studied less frequently (Atha et al., 1985; Sherman et al., 2004; Walilko et al., 2005). Identifying the force exerted by different punches to the head and how the head responds to the punches are important for injury prevention and protective equipment standards. In addition, most boxing related studies focus solely on male participants. With female boxing increasing in popularity, female specific data must be obtained and compared to their male cohorts.

1.2 Background and Significance

Injuries in Boxing

A general injury profile has surfaced from a limited number of studies involving professional and amateur boxers (Timm et al., 1993; Porter and O'Brien, 1996; Zazryn et al., 2003; Zazryn et al., 2006; Zazryn et al., 2009). The most common region of the body for an injury to occur during a competition would be the head/neck/face region

(89 8%) for professional boxers (Zazryn et al, 2003) Over 60% of injuries were classified as open wounds/lacerations generally to the head region (Zazryn et al, 2003, Zazryn et al, 2009) The second most common injury for professional boxers during a competition is a concussion or mild traumatic brain injury (MTBI) (15 9% and 11 7%), followed by fractures occurring less than 10% of the time (Zazryn et al, 2003, Zazryn et al, 2009)

Corresponding injury rates for professional boxers have been published from 25 to 33 injuries per 100 fight participations (Zazryn et al, 2003, Zazryn et al, 2006, Zazryn et al, 2009) Risk factors, such as age and exposure, can increase the risk for injury There is a potential for increased injury risk between the ages of 18 and about 23 and then again from 28 to 35 years of age An increased number of fights will also significantly increase the risk of acute boxing injuries in professional boxers (Zazryn et al, 2009) Taking into account concussions only, the concussion injury rate has been published at 4 per 100 fight participations and 20 8 per 100 fight participations (Zazryn et al, 2003, Zazryn et al, 2006) The data reported in 2006 by Zazryn was collected during 56 fights throughout one year and only recorded 21 injuries Whereas the data reported in 2003 and 2009 were collected over several years and recorded over 100 injuries This could explain higher concussion and injury rates reported in 2006

For amateur competitions the percentage of concussion injuries has been reported from 5 4% to 6 5% (Welch et al, 1986, Jordan et al, 1990) Timm et al (1993) collected injury and illness data over 15 years in athletes who sparred, trained, or competed at the United States Olympic Training Center This study recorded the occurrence of a concussion 74 times or only 6 1% of all injuries While, data collected during training sessions recorded no concussion injuries (Porter and O'Brien, 1996; Zazryn et al., 2006).

The injury rate for amateur boxers was estimated to be 25 per 100 fight participations which is comparable to the injury rates seen in professional boxing (Zazryn et al., 2003; Zazryn et al., 2006; Zazryn et al., 2009). The concussion injury rate for amateur boxers was calculated to be 3.1 per 100 fight participations which is much lower when compared to the rate calculated for professional boxers from the same study, 20.8 per 100 fight participations (Zazryn et al., 2006). With the inconsistency in number of concussions sustained by amateur boxers, the concussion injury rate might be either under or over predicted. While most of the injuries occur during competitions, boxers spend the majority of their time training and very little time actually in competitions (Zazryn et al., 2006).

Although concussions are not as frequent in amateur boxing, studies have found that the repetitive impacts to the head, concussive and sub-concussive, sustained by boxers may generate neurological impairment (Matser et al., 2000; Ng'walali et al., 2000; Warden et al., 2001; Garfield, 2002; Ravdin et al., 2003). Acute injuries in contact and collision sports can result in functional alterations that range from mild traumatic brain injuries (MTBIs or concussions) to death. In the literature, amateur and professional boxers have demonstrated some of the following cognitive dysfunctions: information processing, verbal fluency, planning, attention, memory capacity, and reaction time when compared to baseline testing or controls (Matser et al., 2000; Warden et al., 2001; Ravdin et al., 2003). Acute subdural hematomas are an additional concern to the boxing community because they are potentially fatal. Cases have been identified in the literature of boxers collapsing during a bout due to a subdural hematoma (Ng'walali et al., 2000; Garfield, 2002; Zazryn et al., 2009). Acute injuries occurring from repeated blows to the head can be serious and may lead to a chronic issue.

While severe acute injuries in boxing, including fatalities, are relatively rare compared with other sports (Zazryn et al., 2006), risk of chronic effects of brain injuries in boxing has been documented. Over long periods of time (i.e. over a boxer's career) repeated impacts to the head can lead to chronic traumatic brain injury (also known as chronic traumatic encephalopathy or punch drunk syndrome) (Martland, 1928; Roberts, 1969; Corsellis et al., 1973; Corsellis, 1989; Roberts et al., 1990; McCrory et al., 2007). Researchers have found that professional boxing may lead to chronic traumatic brain injuries (Martland, 1928; Roberts, 1969; Corsellis et al., 1973; Corsellis, 1989; Roberts et al., 1990; Mendez, 1995; Jordan et al., 1997; McCrory et al., 2007). While research indicates that the syndrome is rare and appears in a less severe form in amateur athletes and other contact sports (Haglund and Eriksson, 1993; Moriarity et al., 2004; Loosemore et al., 2007). In addition, researchers have found evidence that the effects of repetitive concussions may be cumulative. Athletes with a history of multiple concussions report more signs and symptoms, demonstrate a lower baseline memory score, and experience a longer recovery period (Collins et al., 1999; Iverson et al., 2003).

Females and Boxing

Although numerous evaluations of both amateur and professional boxers have been completed (Atha et al., 1985; Porter and O'Brien, 1996; Matser et al., 2000; Smith *et al*, 2000, Zazryn *et al*, 2003, Moriarity *et al*, 2004, Sherman *et al*, 2004, Walilko *et al*, 2005, Zazryn *et al*, 2006, Zazryn *et al*, 2009), previous studies have focused solely on male boxers. Even concussion-related studies in other sports frequently do not include female-specific research. One study reviewed the incidence of concussive events for a number of published studies that included both male and female athletes (Hillary *et al*, 2002). Based on the studies included in this analysis, it was determined that the overall concussion incidents per 1000 athletic exposures were 0.35 for females and 0.29 for males. However, when the soccer studies were excluded from analysis it was found that females had an even higher risk of concussion. These studies, which included lacrosse, basketball, and baseball/softball, showed that females had 0.29 concussive events while males had 0.16 concussive events per 1000 athletic exposures (Hillary *et al*, 2002). Additional studies have come to a similar conclusion (Powell and Barber-Foss, 1999, Covassin *et al*, 2003). However, Barnes *et al* and Boden *et al*, concluded that male athletes have a greater risk of concussion when compared to female athletes (Barnes *et al*, 1998, Boden *et al*, 1998). The conflicting data could be attributed to the selection of participants or the design of the studies. One study found that while no neuropsychological differences existed between the male and female high school and collegiate athletes, females reported more symptoms than males (Lovell and West, 2005). Tierney *et al* (2005) studied the gender differences in head-neck segment dynamic stabilization during head acceleration and found females exhibit significantly greater head-neck segment peak angular acceleration despite initiating muscle activity earlier than males (sternocleidomastoid muscle only). The reason for this may be related to females having a lower level of strength, neck girth (30% less), and head neck segment mass (43% less), resulting in less head neck segment stiffness compared to males In the absence of studies focused on the incidence and severity of concussions in those contact sports historically limited to male athletes, a need exists to conduct research of this kind for the female athlete Such results can then be compared to a male cohort in order to determine whether or not gender-related differences exist

While the aforementioned studies included females, the studies did not include athletes from the boxing community Only one study has conducted a medical survey of female boxers (Bianco et al, 2005) This study, however, neglected to include any cognitive evaluation of the females following the bouts Conducting a study including female boxers becomes important as more women participate in this male-dominated sport Recently published articles have reported serious and even fatal injuries to female boxers (Miele et al, 2004, Miele et al, 2006) One recently published case report reviews a female that received a subdural hematoma from boxing (Miele et al, 2004) The clot was removed, however, the boxer experienced neuropsychological difficulties one month after surgery She did not return to the sport of boxing and was in rehabilitation when the article was written Unfortunately, this has not been the most serious injury On April 3, 2005 the first amateur female boxer died after collapsing in the ring following a right hook from her opponent the evening prior to her death The cause of death was a subdural hematoma sustained during the match (Reid, 2005) Both of these cases occurred while the boxers wore protective headgear

The USA Boxing ban on female amateur boxers was officially lifted in 1993 Since that time, there has been an increase in recent years of females in both amateur and professional boxing Approximately 3,000 female boxers register with USA boxing each year, additional research into the forces generated by female boxers and their head response should be conducted (USA Boxing 2009). Therefore, knowledge of cognitive dysfunction, in-ring head accelerations, and differences between genders is critical in establishing gender-specific boxing regulations if needed.

1.3 Specific Aims

Although previously published studies have investigated the punch force generated by amateur boxers, the main focus of these studies were to improve a boxer's technique. More recent studies have begun to investigate the safety concerns that surround this contact sport. In an effort to understand the relationship between forces delivered to the facial region and the risk of head injury, biomechanics of boxer's punches have been studied (Atha et al., 1985; Smith et al., 2000; Sherman et al., 2004; Walilko et al., 2005). However, a variety of mechanical surrogates were used to obtain data in the aforementioned studies. In-ring data collected during practice and competition will provide a more realistic representation of what a boxer experiences. Additionally, male amateur boxers have been the primary focus of previous studies. Female amateur boxing is becoming more popular and gender specific results are needed. The specific aims of this project include:

1. Measure the punch force of punches delivered by male and female amateur boxers using an anthropomorphic surrogate.
2. Measure location, frequency, and severity of impacts sustained by male and female amateur boxers during a sparring session. Assess cognitive function before and after session.

3. Measure location, frequency, and severity of impacts sustained by male and female amateur boxers during a competitive bout. Assess cognitive function before and after bout

CHAPTER 2 - BRAIN INJURY

2.1 Types of Brain Injuries

The brain is composed of soft delicate structures that lie within a rigid skull and is surrounded by a tough outer layer called the dura. Within the brain are cranial nerves that are responsible for many activities such as eye opening, facial movements, speech and hearing. These nerves carry and receive messages that allow the person to think and function normally. However, external forces may cause a tearing and/or twisting of the nerves and blood vessels causing normal function to cease. The result of forces, translational and rotational, generated in the brain caused by rapid acceleration or deceleration is brain injury.

There are two basic types of brain injury that occur: focal and diffuse. Focal injuries typically result from direct mechanical forces producing localized damage to the brain (Hammeke and Gennarelli, 2003). Focal injuries include contusions and hematomas and are most commonly related to direct impacts. A few examples include cerebral contusions and subdural and epidural hematomas. A cerebral contusion is a form of traumatic brain injury (TBI) and is a bruise of the brain tissue caused by small blood vessels leaking into the brain tissue. A subdural hematoma (SDH) is a form of TBI in which blood gathers between the dura mater and the arachnoid membrane. Subdural hematomas are usually caused by the rupture of bridge veins, which allows blood to pool in subdural space. With the dura and arachnoid being well separated, blood can spread freely across the brain surface, increasing intracranial pressure (Auer, 1989). Often there is also significant damage to the underlying brain (contusion or edema). SDHs account for the majority of lethal brain injuries in sports (Bailes and

Cantu, 2001; Cantu and Mueller, 2003). An epidural hematoma (EDH), less common than a subdural, is a type of TBI in which a buildup of blood occurs between the dura and the skull. An epidural bleed is usually the result of tearing arteries. Symptoms include intense headaches and progressive neurological deterioration (Miele *et al.*, 2006). Early recognition and management are essential and complete neurological recovery can be expected.

Diffuse injuries such as a concussion/mild traumatic brain injury (MTBI) or diffuse axonal injuries affect the entire brain and can be more severe. Diffuse injuries are the result of damaging both neurons and blood vessels. An MTBI can be defined as an immediate disturbance of neurological function due to mechanical forces (Symonds, 1962). Diffuse axonal injury (DAI) is caused by the disruption of axons creating lesions in the white matter of the brain (Granacher Jr., 2008). DAI is one of the major causes of unconsciousness and persistent vegetative state following head injury. Like concussions, DAI is the result of shearing forces that occur during rapid acceleration or deceleration, however, DAI can be much more severe. Magnitude of DAI injury depends on the arc of rotation, distance from the center of rotation, and strength and extent of force (Miele *et al.*, 2006).

According to the Center for Disease Control and Prevention (CDC), an MTBI is defined as one or more of the following conditions: "(1) Any period of observed or self-reported transient confusion, disorientation, impaired consciousness, dysfunction of memory around time of injury, or loss of consciousness lasting less than 30 minutes. (2) Observed signs of neurological or neuropsychological dysfunction such as headache, dizziness, irritability, fatigue, or poor concentration"(Gerberding and Binder, 2003).

Injuries that are considered MTBIs or concussions may occur without loss of consciousness. There are several grades of concussion defined in sports. Grade 1 – symptoms resolving in less than 15 minutes with no loss of consciousness and transient confusion, Grade 2 – symptoms resolving in more than 15 minutes with no loss of consciousness and transient confusion, and Grade 3 – loss of consciousness no matter the duration (AAN, 1997).

Participants in most contact sports, such as boxing and football, are at risk for sustaining concussions. In addition, multiple concussions may cause further brain injuries that could include Second Impact Syndrome and cumulative neuropsychological deficits. Second Impact Syndrome (SIS) was first identified by Schneider when he described two athletes who died after a concussion followed by a second minor impact (Schneider, 1973). This condition was better defined in 1984 (Saunders and Harbaugh, 1984). Saunders and Harbaugh (1984) describe an incident where a football player receives a Grade 3 concussion where he lost consciousness. The athlete returned to play and died 4 days later with diffuse cerebral edema.

SIS is thought to occur when an individual sustains a second head injury, usually a concussion, before symptoms associated with the first have subsided. The second impact may be a minor indirect impact imparting accelerative forces to the brain. The athlete will appear stunned but usually does not lose consciousness. What happens in the next 15 seconds to several minutes sets this syndrome apart from a concussion or even a subdural hematoma (Cantu, 1998). Within seconds to minutes of the second impact the athlete collapses to the ground, semicomatose with rapidly dilating pupils, loss of eye movement, and evidence of respiratory failure. Cantu (1998) includes five cases from boxers that illustrated the symptoms of SIS. Although this condition is a concern, fortunately it is a rare occurrence.

In addition to SIS, the cumulative effects of repetitive head injury are a concern in contact sports (Gronwall and Wrightson, 1975, Collins *et al*, 1999, Gaetz *et al*, 2000, Macciocchi *et al*, 2001, Guskiewicz *et al*, 2003, Iverson *et al*, 2003, Iverson *et al*, 2006). A novel study by Gronwall and Wrightson (1975), reported that information processing rapidly decreases after a concussion and the decrease is significantly greater and lasts significantly longer when a history of previous head trauma is noted. Recent studies have supported this conclusion in the athletic population. Athletes with a history of multiple concussions report more signs and symptoms, demonstrate a lower baseline memory score, and experience a longer recovery period (Collins *et al*, 1999, Gaetz *et al*, 2000, Iverson *et al*, 2003). Repeated blows to the head, both sub-concussive and concussive, may lead to chronic traumatic brain injury (also known as punch drunk, chronic traumatic encephalopathy, or dementia pugilistica) (Martland, 1928, Roberts, 1969, Corsellis *et al*, 1973, Corsellis, 1989, Roberts *et al*, 1990, Mendez, 1995, Matser *et al*, 1998, Kutner *et al*, 2000, McCrory *et al*, 2007). Literature supports the fact that chronic brain damage occurs in professional boxers (Martland, 1928, Roberts, 1969, Corsellis *et al*, 1973, Corsellis, 1989, Roberts *et al*, 1990, Mendez, 1995, Jordan *et al*, 1997, McCrory *et al*, 2007), while the literature concerning potential risks for amateur athletes and other contact sports is minimal, the research indicates that the syndrome is rare and appears in a less severe form (Haglund and Eriksson, 1993, Moriarity *et al*, 2004, Loosemore *et al*, 2007).

2.2 Head Injury Mechanism and Injury Prediction

Over the years, a number of studies have been conducted to better understand brain injuries and the mechanism that causes them. There are two main theories of head injuries. The first theory suggests that translational acceleration generated by a direct impact is considered the most important mechanism of head injury (Gurdjian, 1945; Gurdjian *et al.*, 1955; Gurdjian and Lissner, 1961). In 1971 and 1972, Gennarelli and co-workers reported that translational acceleration causes focal injuries, while rotational acceleration causes diffuse brain injuries (Gennarelli *et al.*, 1971; Gennarelli *et al.*, 1972). The second theory suggests that rotational acceleration with or without direct impact should be considered the most important mechanism. Holbourn was the first to propose that translational acceleration would have an insignificant effect and that rotational or angular acceleration would generate maximum shear (Holbourn, 1943). Holbourn suggested the cause of a concussion was due to the shear strain and tensile strain produced by the rotational acceleration. Although, when testing animals, translational and rotational accelerations can individually cause brain injury, there is rarely an impact in the real world that is purely rotational or translational. Therefore, more research is needed to determine the validity of these theories.

The aforementioned studies point to deformation or strain as a primary cause of injury however, these measurements are nearly impossible to obtain in the laboratory. Therefore, variables such as head acceleration are used to characterize the mechanism of injury. Studies have been conducted to determine the rotational acceleration necessary to generate an MTBI. Data derived from experiments by Ommaya *et al.* determine the rotational acceleration required to produce a concussion from whiplash in adults was approximately 1800 rad/s^2 (Ommaya and Hirsch, 1971). Rotational acceleration has been proposed by Lowenhielm as the cause of gliding contusions if a maximum rotational acceleration of 4500 rad/s^2 was achieved (Lowenhielm, 1975). The results yielded by Ommaya et al. (1971) were based on scaling from an animal model.

Two recent studies proposed thresholds for translational and rotational acceleration (King et al., 2003; Zhang et al., 2004). Zhang et al. (2004) used data from football head impact recreations (Newman et al., 2000) and finite element modeling to determine an injury threshold for MTBI. Using data from these recreations as input values, the Wayne State Brain Injury Model was used to determine probability of injury (Zhang et al., 2004). The model was used to calculate the brain's mechanical responses which were then related to an injury severity and the resultant probability of injury. A 25% probability (p = 0.25) of brain injury is 66 g translational and 4,600 rad/s^2 rotational acceleration. A 50% probability (p = 0.50) of brain injury is 82 g and 5,900 rad/s^2 was established for translational and rotational acceleration respectively. An 80% probability (p = 0.80) of brain injury is 106 g of translational acceleration and 7,900 rad/s^2 of rotational acceleration. An additional study proposed much higher thresholds for MTBI (Funk et al., 2007). This study collect head accelerations during collegiate football games using a wireless telemetry system installed in the football helmets. However, only 4 concussive impacts were collected during the duration of this study.

To assess the risk of head injuries, a relationship was developed between impulse duration and acceleration with respect to head injury. This relationship became known as the Wayne State Tolerance Curve (WSTC) and has become the basis of most head-injury tolerance criteria. The WSTC was based on head acceleration data from animal concussion tests and cadaveric skull fractures due to a rigid, flat impact on the forehead. The curve indicated a decrease in the tolerable level of acceleration as pulse duration increased. Because the WSTC had various interpretive difficulties associated with it, C.W. Gadd introduced the Gadd Severity Index (GSI) as a generalization of the Wayne Curve (McElhaney *et al.*, 1976). The severity index may be determined using the following equation:

$$GSI = \int_0^\tau a^{2.5} \, dt$$

Where

a = head acceleration response function
τ = pulse duration
t = integral parameter of time

The slope of the Gadd's log-log plot was -2.5 and 2.5 became the power weighting factor. It was suggested that if the GSI exceeded 1,000, there was a threat to life.

Another parameter was developed by Versace in 1971, the Head Injury Criterion (HIC), based on the WSTC and GSI (Versace, 1971; McElhaney *et al.*, 1976). Backaitis and Eppinger reported that HIC could be interpreted as a measure of the rate of change of specific kinetic energy imparted to the head (Backaitis, 1981; Eppinger, 1981). It is based on the resultant translational acceleration and is determined using the following equation:

$$HIC = [(\frac{1}{t_2 - t_1}) \times \int_{t1}^{t2} a\,dt]^{2.5} (t_2 - t_1)$$

When:

t_1 = an arbitrary time in the pulse
t_2 = for a given t_1, a time in the pulse which maximizes the HIC
a = resultant acceleration at the head center of gravity

The time duration, $t_2 - t_1$ has been proposed include 16 and 36 ms. Prasad and Mertz recommended HIC duration be limited to 15 ms or less (Prasad and Mertz, 1985). Based on their analysis of cadaver data, and using the analysis technique of Mertz and Weber, a HIC of 1000 represented a 16% risk of AIS 4 or greater brain injury (Mertz and Weber, 1982). This value was later set as the Federal Motor Vehicle Safety Standard (FMVSS) 208 standard for frontal automobile accidents. The current FMVSS 208 standard requires the HIC to be less than 700. For the risk prediction of an MTBI, a study proposed a HIC of 250 which is based on reconstructed concussed events from the National Football League (Pellman *et al.*, 2003).

2.3 Diagnostic Tools

In many athletes, concussions go untreated since few symptoms are visible to a casual observer. In addition, athletes frequently do not report symptoms to a trainer or coach due to pressures to remain in the sporting activity which unknowingly could worsen the situation. Developing ways to identify brain injuries have become very important. To help prevent difficulties with concussions, the brain injury must be managed properly using one of the many concussion assessment tools. However, the recognition of a concussion may be difficult for many reasons.

Traumatic brain injuries can be diagnosed using various neuroimaging and laboratory techniques. These techniques include computed tomography of the brain (CT scan), X-rays of the skull, magnetic resonance imaging (MRI), and single photon emission computed tomography (SPECT). Biomarkers, such as S-100 protein, have also been identified to help clinicians determine severity of TBI and the occurrence of an injury (Ingebrigtsen and Rommer, 2002). Although these techniques may be helpful in identifying more serious head injuries, they are not as effective in identifying concussion (De Kruijk *et al.*, 2001).

Neuropsychological tests and assessments can also be used to identify cognitive impairments and to assist in recovery. Tests have been developed to assess cognitive functioning based on memory, learning, motor abilities, attention, and reaction time. These types of tools are employed at the high school, college, and professional levels in order to determine if an injured athlete has suffered neurocognitive impairment during play and to determine when athletes are ready to return to the sport. In the literature, several different types of assessments have been utilized (McCrea *et al.*, 1997; McCrea *et al.*, 1998; McCrea, 2001; Field *et al.*, 2003; Lovell *et al.*, 2004; Lipsky *et al.*, 2005; Terrell *et al.*, 2008). One such tool that has been used to aid in the detection of a concussion in athletes is the Standardized Assessment of Concussion (SAC) (McCrea *et al.*, 1997; McCrea *et al.*, 1998; McCrea, 2001). This test was designed for use on the sideline immediately following a potential concussive impact to clarify the neurocognitive effects of the impact. The SAC requires approximately 5 minutes to administer and tests the athlete's concentration, immediate memory, delayed recall, and orientation. Scores from the baseline test are compared to the scores following the injurious impact.

Concussed athletes score significantly below nonconcussed individuals and below their own baselines SAC score (McCrea et al., 1998).

An alternative option is the concussion recognition and management computerized test, ImPACT© Concussion Management Software. This software can be employed to detect whether an athlete is expressing symptoms of a concussion after an impact and measures an athlete's attention, memory, processing speed, and reaction time via a computerized assessment (ImPACT Applications Inc., 2004). Baseline testing is obtained from the athlete prior to the event or, in some cases, at the beginning of the athletic season. If a concussion is suspected after an impact during play, the athlete repeats the computerized assessment and the results are compared to the baseline in order to determine if a significant difference exists. The symptoms and cognitive function of the athlete following the injury are recorded and will assist coaches and trainers in determining when the athletes may return to athletic activity. This system is currently being used in many high school, collegiate, and professional athletic programs (Iverson et al., 2003; Pellman et al., 2006).

CHAPTER 3

PUNCH FORCE

Portions of this chapter were submitted to:

Stojsih, S., Sherman, D., Dau, N., Boitano, M., Bir, C., 2010. Gender and basic boxing punch type comparisons. Journal of Biomechanics.

3.1 Introduction

It is well-understood that head injuries are an inherent risk in the sport of boxing. Approximately half of the injuries that occur during an amateur boxing competition are concussions (Porter and O'Brien, 1996). The reported concussion rate for professional and amateur boxers are 20.8 and 3.1, respectively, per 100 fights (Zazryn et al., 2006). Although concussions are less frequent in amateur boxing, acute and chronic head injuries are still a concern. Identifying the force exerted by different punches to the head and how the head responds to the punches are important concerns for injury prevention and protective equipment standards.

Several studies have evaluated the biomechanics of a boxer's punch using different surrogate models (Atha et al., 1985; Smith et al., 2000; Walilko et al., 2005). Atha et al. (1985) gathered data from a single world ranked British professional heavy weight boxer using an instrumented target mass suspended as a ballistic pendulum. Smith et al. (2000) developed a boxing dynamometer to measure the force of a cross punch generated by boxers of different experience levels. These surrogate models were developed with a few applications in mind: identifying strengths and weaknesses in technique, allowing coaches to adjust training to obtain a higher punch force, and as a scientific tool to assess the key safety issues in the sport of boxing.

One advanced surrogate, used mainly in automotive safety research, is an anthropomorphic test dummy (ATD). These surrogates were initially developed as an inexpensive way to obtain reproducible results when testing automobiles and aircrafts. One current ATD, the Hybrid III test dummy, is designed to mimic human physical characteristics so that their mechanical responses simulate corresponding human responses. The sports community has utilized this surrogate to obtain head acceleration and injury risk data (Pellman *et al.*, 2003; Sherman *et al.*, 2004; Walilko *et al.*, 2005). Injury criteria have been established to correlate a biomechanical response with a risk of injury. One such criterion used to assess head injury is called the Head Injury Criterion (HIC). Recently, a HIC value of 250 was suggested as a threshold for concussions in professional football (Pellman *et al.*, 2003).

Although the HIC focuses on translational head acceleration, forces produced by rapid acceleration or deceleration of the head can cause both translational and rotational movement of the brain and result in varying levels of injury. A past study conducted by Ommaya and Hirsch (1971) determined the rotational acceleration required to produce a concussion in adults was approximately 1800 rad/s^2. Zhang *et al.* (2004) proposed thresholds for both translational and rotational acceleration based on a finite element model of the brain. The model established that translational and rotational acceleration of 66 *g* and 4600 rad/s^2 (25% probability), 82 *g* and 5900 rad/s^2 (50% probability), and 106 *g* and 7900 rad/s^2 (80% probability), respectively, would result in brain injury.

The first utilization of the Hybrid III in boxing research was by Walilko *et al.* (2005) who used a standard 50th percentile male Hybrid III (Denton ATD, Inc) to collect head acceleration and injury risk data from a cross punch to the jaw. Data were collected from seven Olympic boxers. In a follow up study, Sherman *et al.* (2004) collected punch force and injury criterion data from 11 boxers evaluating four different boxing punches. Although these studies have evaluated the biomechanics of common boxing punches, the focus has been on male athletes. Female boxing, both amateur and professional, has increased in popularity and should also be considered.

A recent study by Stojsih *et al.* (2008) collected in-ring head acceleration data from 30 female and 30 male amateur boxers during sparring sessions. Each participant wore an instrumented headgear during a practice bout and the head acceleration, injury criterion, duration, and location were recorded for each impact. This is the first study that has investigated the biomechanics of female boxers. With the increasing popularity of women's boxing, approximately 3000 female boxers register with USA boxing each year, additional research into the forces generated by female boxers and their head response is recommended (USA Boxing 2009).

The current effort was conducted to study and compare the biomechanics of three main boxing punch types for both male and female Olympic-level boxers. The goal was to identify any differences between the genders in terms of hand velocity, punch force, head acceleration and injury criterion using the Hybrid III ATD. In addition, the different punch types were compared.

3.2 Methodology

Test Setup

A total of 75 Olympic-level and amateur boxers (18 – 34 years of age) participated in this study, conducted during the USA Boxing National Competition at the

Olympic Training Center in Colorado Springs, Colorado and the Ringside World Championship in Kansas City, Missouri. Anthropomorphic details are provided in Table 3.1. Approval was granted by the Wayne State University Human Investigation Committee prior to the study.

Table 3.1: Descriptive characteristics of sample population

	N	Height (in.)	Weight (lbs.)
Female	15	66±3	141±25
Male	60	69±3	159±37

Each boxer was asked to throw three main boxing punch types (hook, jab, and cross) in their normal manner at a Hybrid III headform. Boxers were given a chance to practice prior to data collection. If a punch did not connect with the headform or the punch was not positioned correctly, the boxer was asked to repeat the punch. A hook punch begins with the lead hand brought from the side towards the center of the temporal region, swinging from the shoulder with the arm bent. A jab is a quick, cross punch with the lead hand aimed at the center of the head. A cross punch is thrown with the rear hand, pre-positioned at the chin, and landing at the opponent's chin with the fist traveling in a straight line. For this study, lead punches were performed with the participants' non-dominant hand and rear punches were performed with the dominant hand. Punch force, hand velocity, head acceleration, for each punch was determined and injury criterion was measured. Data for the different punch types were then compared.

The study methodology followed a testing protocol similar to previous studies, with the addition of female boxers (Sherman *et al.*, 2004; Walilko *et al.*, 2005). A 50th percentile male Hybrid III ATD headform with a frangible face, connected to the neck and torso to ensure realistic headform motion, was used. The apparatus was secured to a table which was adjusted to the participant's height, ensuring they delivered horizontal punches. The frangible face improves the biofidelity of the surrogate during facial impacts and reduces the risk of injury to the striking fist. Certified headgear was placed on the headform and was properly adjusted prior to each impact. Although the Hybrid III neck was used for this study, it is unknown whether the neck precisely characterizes the boxing population since their neck muscles may be stronger than the average population due to specialized training.

Instrumentation

A tri-axial block of Endevco (San Juan Capistrano, CA) 7264-2K accelerometers in an orthogonal array was secured inside boxer's palm using handwrap prior to donning the glove. Nine additional Endevco (San Juan Capistrano, CA) 7264-2k accelerometers were mounted in the headform in a 3-2-2-2 array (Padgaonkar *et al.*, 1975). A six-axis upper neck loadcell (Denton, ATD, Rochester Hills, MI) was used to measure neck loads and moments. The primary data acquisition system was the TDAS PRO (DTS, Inc. Seal Beach, CA). Data were collected at a sampling rate of 10 KHz and post processed according to SAE J211-1 (SAE, 1995).

Calculation of Head Linear and Angular Acceleration

Translational accelerations at the headform center of gravity (CG) were used to calculate HIC value for each punch. The formula used for calculation is indicated below:

$$HIC = [(\frac{1}{t2-t1}) \times \int_{t1}^{t2} adt]^{2.5} (t2 - t1) \qquad (1)$$

Where, in practice, $t_2 - t_1$ is a rolling 15 ms span and a is the resultant translational acceleration at the head center of gravity.

Rotational acceleration of the headform was calculated using the 3-2-2-2 method (Padgaonkar et al., 1975). This method takes into account differences in acceleration measured in four locations on a rigid body to derive rotational acceleration about an axis.

Calculation of Punch Force

Impact force applied by the boxer was determined using data from the upper neck load cell and acceleration at the CG of the headform as previously described (Walilko et al., 2005). The resultant value for punch force was determined based on data from all three axes. The equations of motion used for each axis are:

$$Fp_x - Fn_x = ma_x \quad (3)$$

$$Fp_y - Fn_y = ma_y \quad (4)$$

$$Fp_z - Fn_z = ma_z \quad (5)$$

Where Fp_n is the force applied to the headform by the boxer in the n direction, Fn_n is the neck shear force, m is the mass of headform and a_n is the n direction translational acceleration at the headform CG. The resultant value for the punch force was calculated by:

$$Fp = ((ma_x)^2 + (ma_y)^2 + (ma_z)^2)^{.5} \quad (6)$$

Hand Velocity

Hand velocity was determined by integrating the resultant hand acceleration up to face contact. Face contact was determined by the rapid change in resultant acceleration. This technique was previously validated against video data and showed correlation between the two velocity measurements (Walilko et al., 2005).

3.3 Statistics

Biomechanical punch data were analyzed using Statistical Package for Social Sciences (SPSS) version 16.0.2. A MANOVA was conducted when comparing the dependent variables for the genders; however, violations of normality and variance occurred and a non-parametric test (Mann-Whitney) was used to make comparisons. The Kruskal-Wallis test was conducted to compare the dependent variables to the punch types within both genders. If there was a statistically significant difference the punch types were then compared using a Mann-Whitney test. Since the sample population was small for the female boxers, Exact One Way ANOVA (STATA Statistics/Data Analysis Software) was used to verify results and determine if the result was an effect of low power. The independent variables included: gender, punch type, and weight class. The dependent variables consisted of: head acceleration, hand velocity, punch force, and injury criterion. A Pearson Correlation test was used to compare the anthropomorphic data and experimental data. The Pearson Correlations were administered separately for the male and female data. While the male data were separated by punch type, the female data were not since no significant difference was detected between punch types. Alpha level was set at $p < 0.05$ and 2-tailed significance values are listed.

3.4 Results

Evaluation of boxers

A total of 143 punches were included in the study. The number and punch types varied for each individual. These include 44 hooks (34 male, 10 female), 43 jabs (33 male, 10 female), and 56 crosses (46 male, 10 female). The data were categorized and analyzed by gender and punch type. Comparing the data by weight class was not possible since weight classes are defined differently for male and female boxers. In addition, the weight class data could not be compared within genders since the number of participants in each weight class was too small.

Calculated Punch Force and Biomechanical Responses

The mean punch force and hand velocity were separated by punch type and gender (Table 3.2). The overall mean punch force for the female boxers was 1488±840 N and the overall mean punch force for the male boxers was 2433±1489 N. Without taking into account punch type, male boxers had a significantly higher punch force ($p < 0.01$) when compared to the female data using the Mann-Whitney test. The overall mean hand velocity for the female athletes was significantly lower at 8±2 m/s than the mean hand velocity for males at 10±3 m/s ($p < 0.01$). The relationship between force and weight was determined by Pearson's correlation, which measures the association between variables.

Table 3.2. Mean punch force and hand velocity for each punch type by gender († p < 0.05 when comparing genders, ‡ p < 0.05 when comparing punches within gender, and ‡* indicates that the hand velocity is not significantly different when comparing the jab and cross)

	Punch Type	N	Punch Force (N)	Hand Velocity (m/s)
FEMALE	Hook	10	1776±559	9±2
	Jab	10	1417±605	8±2
	Cross	10	1270±1203	7±1
	Overall Mean†	**30**	**1488±840**	**8±2**
MALE	Hook‡	34	3431±1269	11±3
	Jab‡	33	2487±1167	9±3
	Cross‡*	46	1656±1414	9±1
	Overall Mean†	**113**	**2433±1489**	**10±3**

Comparing three punch types for the female boxers, using a Kruskal-Wallis test, showed no significant difference in punch force (p = 0.179) or hand velocity (p = 0.258) (Table 3.2). These results were verified using an exact significance test. Although, the power was lower than desired the exact test supported the results from the Kruskal-Wallis test. For male boxers, all three punches were significantly different from one another when comparing punch force (Table 3.2). The hook generated a significantly higher punch force when compared to the jab and cross (p < 0.01) and the jab generated a higher force when compared to the cross (p < 0.01). Comparing the velocity data determined that the hook was significantly greater than both the jab and cross (p < 0.01).

Resultant Head Acceleration and Injury Criterion

Mean head acceleration for the headform CG and injury criterion were collected or calculated for each punch type and gender (Figure 3.1 and Table 3.3). Overall mean translational headform acceleration generated by females and males were 29±14 g's and 49±23 g's, respectively. Overall mean rotational headform acceleration generated by female boxers was 3062±1268 rad/s^2 and by males was 5322±3010 rad/s^2. Overall mean HIC values were 16±16 for female boxers and 54±52 for the male boxers. The Mann-Whitney test was used to compare the mean headform head acceleration and HIC values between genders and it was found that the head accelerations generated by the male athletes and HIC values were significantly higher ($p < 0.01$) when compared to the values produced by females.

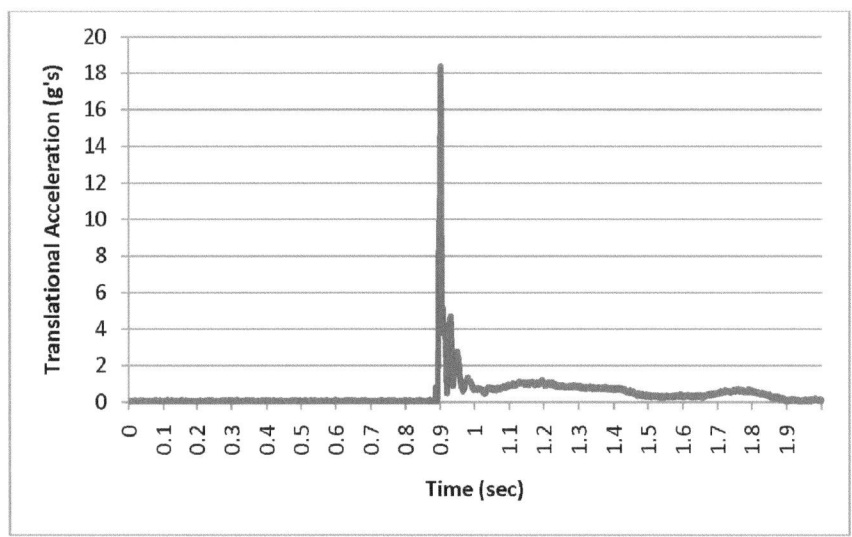

Figure 3.1: Example of head acceleration data collected from the HIII

Table 3.3: Mean head acceleration and injury criterion for each punch by gender († p < 0.05 when comparing genders, ‡ p < 0.05 when comparing punches within gender, and ‡* indicates that the head acceleration is not significantly different when comparing the jab and cross)

	Punch Type	N	Trans. Accel. (g)	Rot. Accel. (rad/s^2)	HIC
FEMALE	Hook	10	34±14	3156±831	17±11
	Jab	10	22±11	2762±970	9±9
	Cross	10	30±15	3269±1842	21±23
	Overall Mean†	**30**	**29±14**	**3062±1268**	**16±16**
MALE	Hook‡	34	62±26	6440±2825	77±69
	Jab‡	33	41±22	4927±1863	42±50
	Cross‡*	46	45±15	4779±3588	46±29
	Overall Mean†	**113**	**49±23**	**5322±3010**	**54±52**

The Kruskal-Wallis test was used to compare head acceleration and injury criterion produced by different types of punches within genders. No statistical significance was found when analyzing translational acceleration ($p = 0.119$), rotational acceleration ($p = 0.606$), and HIC ($p = 0.232$) for each punch type produced by female boxers (Table 3.3). These results were also verified by an exact significance test. Again, for male boxers, all three punches were significantly different from one another when comparing HIC values (Table 3.3). The hook generated a significantly higher HIC when compared to the jab and cross ($p < 0.02$) and the cross generated a higher HIC when compared to the jab ($p < 0.01$). The hook punch generated a significantly higher headform head acceleration ($p < 0.02$) when compared to both the jab and cross punches. However, there was no significant difference between the jab and the cross punches ($p > 0.05$) when comparing head acceleration.

A weak linear relationship existed when comparing anthropomorphic data to head acceleration of the headform, punch force, and HIC for the female boxers (Table

3.4). The highest r-value was found between weight and rotational acceleration at r = 0.575 and although this comparison is statistically significant it is still considered a weak positive linear relationship. A weak linear relationship also existed when analyzing the male data. The only punch having statistical significance was the jab punch. Although there was statistical significance, similar to the female data, the positive linear correlations when comparing weight to punch force, head accelerations, and HIC proved to be weak (Table 3.5). For both male and female boxers, the punch force has a strong correlation with HIC. This finding coincides with previously published literature (Sherman *et al.*, 2004; Walilko *et al.*, 2005).

Table 3.4: Correlations between punch dynamics and risk of injury parameters for female athletes (‡ $p < 0.05$ and ‡‡ $p < 0.01$)

	Weight	Height	Rot. Accel.	Trans. Accel.	Punch Force	Hand Velocity	HIC
Weight	1	0.824‡‡	0.575‡‡	0.446‡	0.461‡	-0.177	0.473‡‡
Height	0.824‡‡	1	0.457‡	0.287	0.387‡	-0.180	0.321
Rot. Accel.	0.575‡‡	0.457‡	1	0.732‡‡	0.842‡‡	0.308	0.781‡‡
Trans. Accel.	0.446‡	0.287	0.732‡‡	1	0.812‡‡	0.488‡‡	0.897‡‡
Punch Force	0.461‡	0.387	0.842‡‡	0.812‡‡	1	0.490‡‡	0.807‡
Hand Velocity	-0.177	-0.180	0.308	0.488‡‡	0.490‡‡	1	0.339
HIC	0.473‡‡	0.321	0.781‡‡	0.897‡‡	0.807‡‡	0.339	1

Table 3.5: Correlations between punch dynamics and risk of injury parameters for male athletes generated by the jab punch (‡ p < 0.05 and ‡‡ p < 0.01)

	Weight	Height	Rot. Accel.	Trans. Accel.	Punch Force	Hand Velocity	HIC
Weight	1	0.686‡‡	0.494‡‡	0.510‡‡	0.531‡‡	0.214	0.521‡‡
Height	0.686‡‡	1	0.519‡‡	0.592‡‡	0.606‡‡	0.305	0.604‡‡
Rot. Accel.	0.494‡‡	0.519‡‡	1	0.750‡‡	0.793‡‡	0.254	0.669‡‡
Trans. Accel.	0.510‡‡	0.592‡‡	0.750‡‡	1	0.991‡‡	0.641‡‡	0.964‡‡
Punch Force	0.531‡‡	0.606‡‡	0.793‡‡	0.991‡‡	1	0.620‡‡	0.947‡‡
Hand Velocity	0.214	0.305	0.254	0.641‡‡	0.620‡‡	1	0.620‡‡
HIC	0.521‡‡	0.604‡‡	0.669‡‡	0.964‡‡	0.947‡‡	0.620‡‡	1

3.5 Discussion

The goal of the current study was to determine the biomechanics of three different punches and compare values from male and female boxers. The Hybrid III was used as a surrogate since it closely represents the mass and response of the average human head and neck. Punch force, hand velocity, head acceleration, and injury criterion were collected.

The current study collected data from three different boxing punches, while, previous studies have focused primarily on one particular punch. Table 3.6 compares the values recorded by three previous studies to the current study. Smith *et al.* (2000) recorded the punch force generated from a jab and cross punch delivered by 23 male boxers (elite, intermediate, and novice) using a dynamometer. These data compare well with the current study for the jab. However, the cross punch seemed to generate higher values than those collected for this study.

Walilko et al. (2005) evaluated a cross punch to the jaw using the 50th percentile Hybrid III male dummy. Punch force, head acceleration, and HIC values were slightly higher when compared to data from the current study. In this previous study, weight was found to increase linearly with punch force, rotation head acceleration, and HIC. In the current study, this was not the case. The cross and hook punch types did not demonstrate a linear relationship between dependent and independent variables. However, the jab proved to have linear relationships when comparing weight with head acceleration, punch force, and HIC.

Additionally, Sherman et al. (2004) collected data from 11 Olympic-level boxers using the 50th percentile Hybrid III male dummy. When comparing cross and hook punch biomechanical data, the athletes in the current study generated lower punch force values but comparable HIC values.

Table 3.6: Comparison of biomechanical data found in literature

Punch Type	Study	Punch Force (N)	Hand Velocity (m/s)	Trans. Accel. (g)	Rot. Accel. (rad/s^2)	HIC
JAB	Current	2487±1167	-	-	-	-
	Smith et al.					
	Elite	2847±596	-	-	-	-
	Intermediate	2283±355	-	-	-	-
	Novice	1604±273	-	-	-	-
CROSS	Current	1656±1414	9±1	45±15	4779±3588	46±29
	Walilko et al.	3427±811	9.14±2.06	58±13	6343±1789	71±49
	Sherman et al.	2284±951	-	-	-	55±43
	Smith et al.					
	Elite	4800±227	-	-	-	-
	Intermediate	3722±133	-	-	-	-
	Novice	2381±116	-	-	-	-
HOOK	Current	3431±1269	-	-	-	77±69
	Sherman et al.	4360±2330	-	-	-	82±69

The hook produced the highest head acceleration for the headform at the CG, 6440±2825 rad/s². Zhang *et al.* (2004) suggested translational and rotational head acceleration thresholds for assessing risk of concussions. The majority of impacts recorded during this study were below the suggested thresholds (Zhang *et al.*, 2004) (Figure 3.2 and 3.3). Combining the data, 83% of the impacts generated translational head acceleration values below the 25% probability of an MTBI. For rotational acceleration, 83% of impacts were below tolerance level.

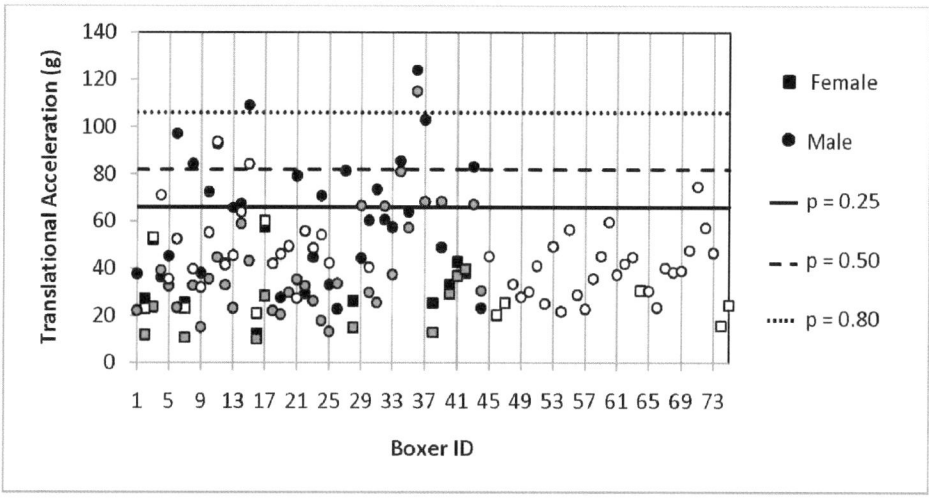

Figure 3.2: Translational headform accelerations produced by female and male athletes (hook-black, jab-grey, and cross-white)

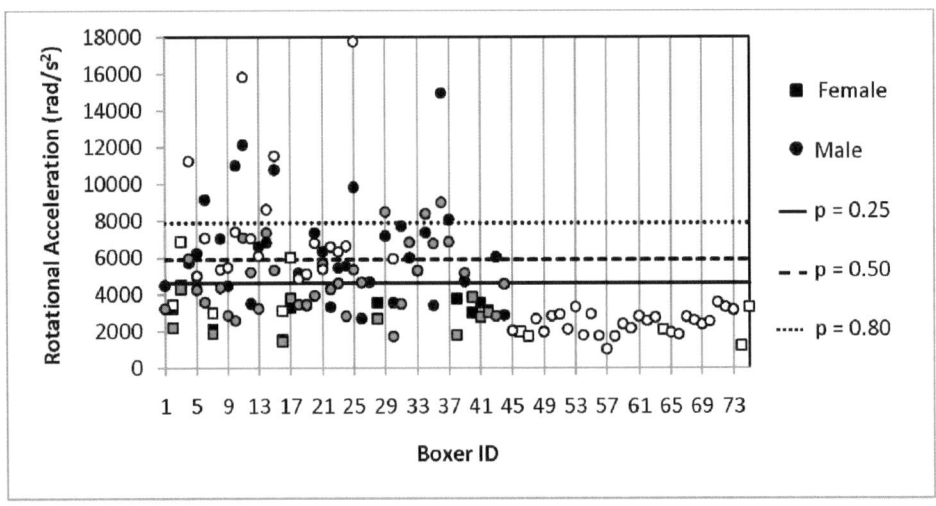

Figure 3.3: Rotational headform acceleration produced by female and male athletes (hook-black, jab-grey, and cross-white)

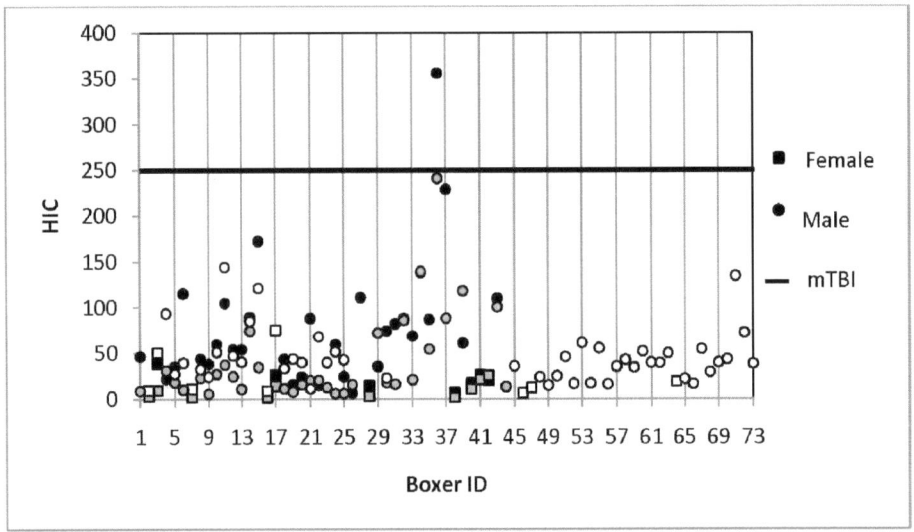

Figure 3.4: HIC values produced by female and male athletes (hook-black, jab-grey, and cross-white)

The HIC value is an additional parameter that is used to predict possible head injury (Figure 3.4). In a study conducted by Pellman *et al.* (2003), MTBI threshold of 250 was established for the HIC values. There was only one impact that exceeded this threshold, therefore, the majority of the punches delivered by boxers are considered sub-concussive. While one sub-concussive impact may not cause a concussion, multiple sub-concussive impacts may cause acute and chronic brain injuries (Martland, 1928, Roberts, 1969, Corsellis et al, 1973, Corsellis, 1989, Roberts et al, 1990, McCrory et al, 2007). In addition, researchers have found evidence that the effects of repetitive concussions may be cumulative. Athletes with a history of multiple concussions report more signs and symptoms, demonstrate a lower baseline memory score, and experience a longer recovery period (Collins et al, 1999, Iverson et al, 2003).

Unfortunately, the array of athletes that were recruited covered a variety of weight classes and although each gender is divided into the same categories, the specifications differ. Male weight divisions range from 106 lb – 201+ lb, while the female weight divisions range from 101 lb – 178+ lb (USA Boxing, 2008). Statistical analyses between genders with respect to weight class could not be performed for this reason. Statistical analyses were attempted to determine if there were any significant differences within gender, however, the number of impacts for each weight division was too small to determine significance. Table 3.7 lists the biomechanical data for each weight class and gender (weight classes are listed in ascending order).

Table 3.7: Mean biomechanical data classification by weight class

	Weight Class	Number of Impacts	Punch Force (N)	Hand Velocity (m/s)	Trans. Accel. (g)	Rot. Accel. (rad/s^2)	HIC
FEMALE	Bantam	1	432	8	31	2081	19
	Feather	8	1236±712	9±2	23±12	2479±922	10±9
	Light	5	1715±799	10±2	33±6	3253±349	17±6
	Welter	3	1325±323	7±2	21±8	2958±661	7±4
	Middle	5	848±574	6±0.3	20±7	1978±652	8±4
	Light Heavy	2	1439±458	11±1	21±8	3103±617	9±8
	Heavy	3	2378±948	9±9	49±18	4349±1462	39±32
	Super Heavy	3	2503±826	7±1	43±17	5225±1447	33±21
MALE	Light Fly	3	2426±740	12±4	44±15	3735±2129	38±31
	Bantam	7	2592±1499	9±3	49±24	5787±2424	39±35
	Feather	11	2293±1249	10±2	46±19	5122±2804	38±20
	Light	8	2285±1215	11±4	44±20	4213±1220	42±35
	Light Welter	13	1687±1214	9±1	38±17	3963±1797	38±30
	Welter	29	2770±1687	10±3	54±25	6174±3357	61±53
	Middle	7	1427±1425	9±2	48±17	4109±2625	52±41
	Light Heavy	11	1586±830	9±2	33±10	3755±1181	26±15
	Heavy	10	3396±1922	11±3	66±36	8565±4746	114±110
	Super Heavy	14	3022±1177	10±3	56±16	5239±2188	73±28

The results collected from the current study for the female boxers are potentially under predicting what is actually occurring in the ring. Stojsih *et al.* (2008) collected biomechanical data from both male and female amateur boxers during sparring. The study collected data using a telemetry system with instrumented headgear. The mean head acceleration data from the headform CG and HIC from the current study were

29±14 g, 3062±1268 rad/s^2, and 16±16, respectively. The mean head acceleration and HIC obtained from sparring were 28±17 g, 2533±1524 rad/s^2, and 32±66, respectively (Stojsih et al., 2008). Although the mean accelerations are similar for the two studies, the head injury criterion values were larger for the sparring data. In the current study, there were 30 impacts analyzed and the peak HIC value was 75. Stojsih et al. (2008) collect data from 83 impacts and the peak HIC was 1079. The range of data collected during sparring and the larger sample population could partially explain the differences in results.

The current study used a Hybrid III 50th male head, neck, and torso for all participants. The 50th male dummy was created based on gender specific anthropomorphic and biomechanical data that was available. The average male head circumference, head weight, and neck girth is larger when compared with females. One study found females exhibited a higher head-neck segment angular acceleration when compared to males (Tierney et al., 2005). The reason for the greater angular acceleration in females may be due to their lower levels of strength, neck girth, and head mass, resulting in less head-neck segment stiffness compared with males. If the neck used in this study had a higher compliance mimicking the actual response of the female neck, angular accelerations and injury criterion values would have increased (Rousseau and Hoshizaki, 2009). Also, in general, the Hybrid III is a standardized testing device that was developed for head-on automobile crash tests and can only approximate how the head will respond to a low velocity impact. While this is not an ideal method for testing boxing punches, the Hybrid III is an inexpensive and reproducible means of collecting sports impact data.

This study quantifies three primary punches in boxing for both male and female amateur boxers. The data collected during this study can be helpful in manufacturing protective equipment. Insight into accelerations and forces caused by different punches may help develop standards for boxing headgear and gloves. Since this study only looked at three maximum punches per athlete, future studies could look into numerous punches, such as those seen in a competitive setting. Also, correlating the head accelerations experienced during multiple punches and the athletes' cognitive function would better define the mechanics of head injuries in boxing.

CHAPTER 4 – BIOMECHANICS OF SPARRING

Portions of this chapter were published in:

Stojsih, S., Boitano, M., Wilhelm, M., Bir, C., 2008. A prospective study of punch biomechanics and cognitive function for amateur boxers. Br J Sports Med, bjsm.2008.052845. (Appendix B)

4.1 Introduction

Although injuries and the mechanisms that cause the injuries in both professional and amateur boxing have been well documented (Atha et al., 1985; Porter and O'Brien, 1996; Smith et al., 2000; Zazryn et al., 2003; Sherman et al., 2004; Bianco et al., 2005; Walilko et al., 2005; Zazryn et al., 2006; Zazryn et al., 2009), head acceleration data from the ring have yet to be obtained. In addition, the correlation of these data to post-bout cognitive function has not been explored.

Several studies have evaluated the biomechanics of a punch using different surrogate models (Atha et al., 1985; Smith et al., 2000; Sherman et al., 2004; Walilko et al., 2005; Stojsih et al., 2010). Atha et al. (1985) gathered data from a world ranked British professional heavyweight boxer using an instrumented target mass suspended as a ballistic pendulum. The maximum translational acceleration recorded was 53 g's, peak contact force was 4096 N, and velocity upon impact was 8.9 m/s. However, the objective of the study was to determine the force of a boxer's punch, not to observe the effects of the punch force in creating an injurious effect. The use of a ballistic pendulum provides force data but does not correlate to head injury risk.

To assess the risk of head injuries due to blunt impact, a relationship has been developed between impulse duration and acceleration. This relationship is commonly known as the Wayne State Tolerance Curve (WSTC) and has become the basis of most head-injury tolerance criteria. The curve indicated a decrease in the tolerable level of acceleration as pulse duration increased. Because the WSTC had various interpretive difficulties associated with it, the Gadd Severity Index (GSI) was introduced as a generalization of the WSTC (Gadd, 1966). A further refinement occurred in 1971 when Versace developed the Head Injury Criterion (HIC), based on the WSTC and GSI (Versace, 1971; McElhaney et al., 1976). Backaitis (1981) and Eppinger (1981) reported that HIC could be interpreted as a measure of the rate of change of specific kinetic energy imparted to the head and is based on the resultant translational acceleration. The well-established HIC threshold of 1000 was developed to identify severe head injuries in automotive safety testing (Gadd, 1966; Versace, 1971). Recently, a HIC value of 250 was suggested as a threshold for MTBI in professional football (Pellman et al., 2003).

Although the HIC focuses on translational acceleration, forces produced by rapid acceleration or deceleration of the head can cause both translational and rotational movement of brain and result in varying levels of injury. A recent study by Zhang et al. (2004) proposed thresholds for both translational and rotational acceleration based on a finite element model of the brain. The threshold established that translational and rotational acceleration of 66 g's and 4,600 rad/s^2 (25% probability), 82 g's and 5,900 rad/s^2 (50% proablility), and 106 g's and 7,900 rad/s^2 (80% probability), respectively, would result in brain injury.

In one of the first studies correlating these injury parameters to impacts from Olympic boxers, Walilko et al. (2005) evaluated the biomechanics of a punch to the jaw and the risk of head injury from translational and rotational accelerations using a Hybrid III anthropomorphic head. The headform provided the ability to not only determine punch force, but to predict the risk of head injury based on the instrumentation and study design. The translational acceleration was reported to be 58±13 g's, rotational acceleration was 6343±1789 rad/s^2, and HIC was 71±49. Although it provides some preliminary data, this study is limited due to the lack of biofidelity of the jaw and Hybrid III headform for such an application.

Given advances in wireless technology, the collection of in-ring data without interference of the play of the game is now possible (Duma *et al.*, 2005; Brolinson *et al.*, 2006). The use of such technology within the sport of boxing will allow for more precise analyses of both the impact and resulting outcome. The goal of the current study was to collect in-ring head acceleration data from amateur boxers and document any resulting cognitive changes.

4.2 Methods

Sample Population

Kelly Air Force Base Testing - 2006

In February 2006, the Armed Forces held a training camp in San Antonio, Texas, for both male and female amateur boxers in preparation for the Armed Forces Boxing Competition. A total of 12 boxers participated in the study, of which 8 were male and 4 were female. Female participants ranged in age from 22 to 28, with experience levels spanning from a minimum of 1 year to a maximum of 5 years at the amateur level. Male participants ranged in age from 21 to 27 with a maximum of 5 years of experience at the amateur level.

Kelly Air Force Base Testing - 2007

A return visit was made to San Antonio for the Armed Forces Competition in March 2007. A total of 2 female amateur boxers consented to participate in the study during the tournament. Participants were 22 and 26 years of age and both have been competing at the amateur level for at least 2 years.

San Antonio, Texas Testing

While in San Antonio for the Armed Forces Competition two local gyms agreed to participate in the study. From one of the gyms, Ramos Boxing Gym, the consent to participate was received from 2 females. The participants were 19 and 23 years of age. One of the females had been boxing at the amateur level for 8 years and the other had been boxing for 1 year. The second gym, Zarzamora Street Gym, also had two female boxers consent. The participants were 23 and 29 with 1 year of experience boxing at the amateur level.

University of Michigan Testing

In March 2007, seven subjects consented to participate in the study from the boxing club at the University of Michigan. This group consisted of 5 female boxers and 2 male boxers. Female participants ranged in age from 19 to 22 with a maximum experience level of 3 years. Male participants were 28 and 30 years of age with a maximum experience level of 3 years.

Olympic Training Center Testing

In April 2007, thirteen subjects consented to participate while attending a boxing training camp at the Olympic Training Center in Colorado Springs, Colorado. This group was comprised of all male boxers. The participants ranged in age from 18 to 25 and the majority had at least 10 years boxing experience at the amateur level. Only 2 of the participants had less than 3 years boxing experience. A return trip was made to the Olympic Training Center in September 2007. This group comprised of 12 female and 7 male amateur boxers. The female participants ranged in age from 18 to 32 with a maximum experience level of 7 years in amateur boxing. Male participants range in age from 18 to 22 with experience levels ranging from 1 to 12 years.

Windsor, Canada Testing

In September 2007, three female subjects consented to participate from two different boxing gyms in Windsor, Ontario. Two of the female boxers train at the Windsor Boxing Club while the other participant trains at the Border City Boxing Gym. The participants ranged in age from 23 to 33 with an experience level of at least 4 years at the amateur level.

Based on all of these sites, a total of 30 male and 30 female amateur boxers were enrolled into the study. The age range for the athletes was 18 to 33 with mean age of 23 and an average experience at the amateur level of 4.5 years. The mean age for the male athletes was 22 years of age with an average experience level of 6.4 years. The mean age for the female athletes was 24 years of age with an average experience of 3 years at the amateur level. Approval was garnered from the Wayne State University Human Investigation Committee prior to testing with all subjects consenting to participate prior to testing.

IBH System

In an effort to collect in-ring peak head accelerations, Simbex Inc. (Lebanon, NH) developed the Instrumented Boxing Headgear (IBH) system (Figures 4.1 and 4.2).

Using this headgear, the translational and rotational accelerations, HIC, GSI, and hit location were determined for each punch (Beckwith *et al.*, 2007)

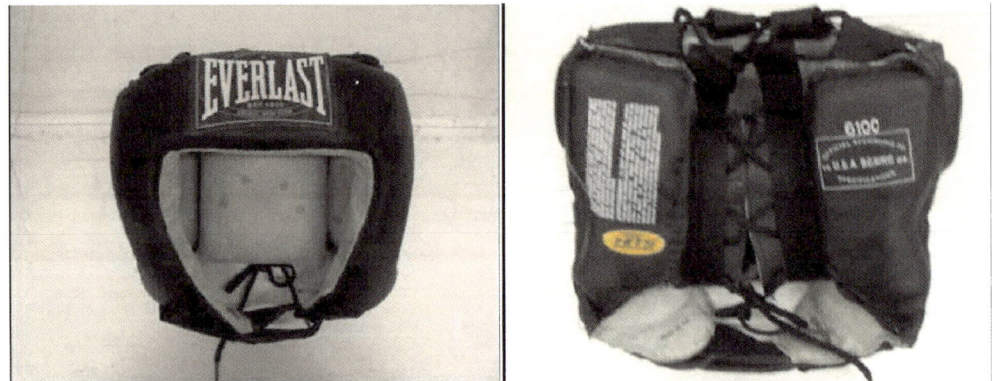

Figure 4.1: Instrumented Boxing Headgear (IBH)

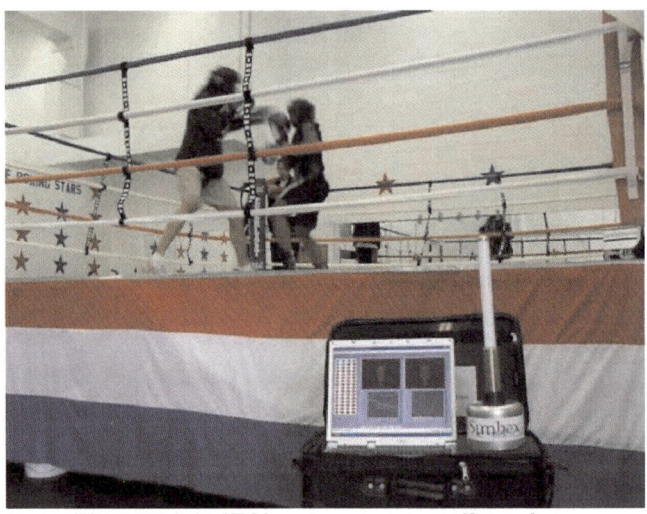

Figure 4.2: IBH system recording data

The IBH system is designed after the Head Impact Telemetry System (HITS) which Simbex developed for use in football helmets. The only difference between the two systems is the amount of single-axis accelerometers mounted in the helmet or headgear. The accelerometers were placed in an array in between the head-side leather and padding of the headgear's backside and rear pads. Placement of the accelerometers was inspired by the need to minimize the probability of direct contact from an impact during the spar. The battery pack and radio were inserted into the rear panel of the headgear between the outside leather and foam pad. The accelerometers, battery, and data acquisition and radio hardware increase headgear weight by only 4 oz.

Each headgear is considered one unit and the data from that unit were transferred via radio frequency to a wireless receiver and laptop computer system. For each impact the time, linear acceleration, rotational acceleration, GSI, and HIC were downloaded to the on-board memory. After the baseline test is completed, the boxers spar for 4-two minute rounds with an opponent of comparable weight and of the same gender. During the sparring the instrumented headgear was worn by one or both of the boxers. Real-time data was downloaded throughout the four rounds. Once the data were collected from the 12 accelerometers, processing was completed by researchers at Simbex, Inc. The peak linear head acceleration, peak rotational head acceleration, HIC, and GSI were established for each impact.

The algorithm that was developed to analyze the HITS data, 6DOF, with only 6 single axis accelerometers is also valid for the IBH data that has 12 single axis accelerometers (Chu et al., 2006; Beckwith et al., 2007). This algorithm computes x, y, and z components of translational and rotational acceleration. The sensing axis of the accelerometers is tangential to the heads surface. Beckwith (2007) validated the IBH system and the algorithm by comparing the results to the HIII acceleration data. Peak linear (r^2 = 0.91) and rotational (r^2 = 0.91) acceleration measures were correlated between IBH and HIII using linear regression (Figure 4.3).

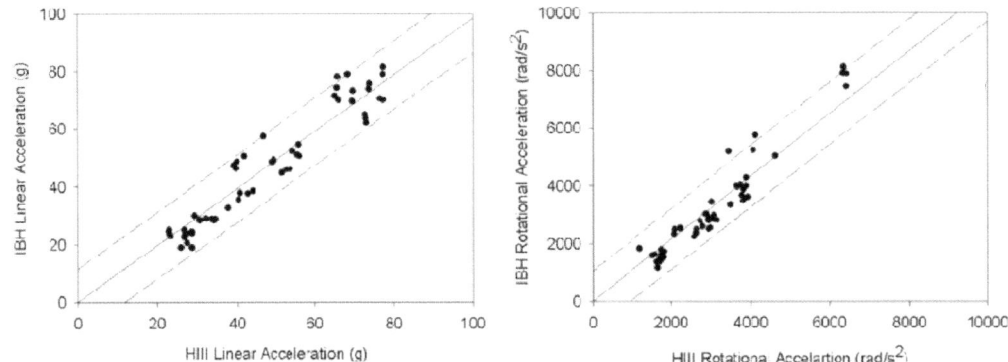

Figure 4.3: Linear regression of IBH acceleration data and HIII 3-2-2-2 acceleration data (Beckwith *et al.*, 2007)

Regression analysis shows that the IBH under predicts HIII peak linear acceleration by 2% and over predicts HIII peak rotational acceleration by 8%. The impact location is detected based on the direction of the impact. The general locations recorded by the IBH were accurate within 1.27 cm, which is believed to be sufficient to document impact location on the head without video. Absolute errors in the computation of injury tolerance metrics HIC and GSI were both 19 ±12%. Differences here were driven by differences in absolute measures of linear acceleration and small variations in the resultant waveform shape at the tails of the impact (Beckwith *et al.*, 2007).

Impacts were grouped into five sections (front, back, top, right, and left) based on the impact location, which is defined by the azimuth (Θ) and elevation (α) of each impact (Figure 4.4). The azimuth (Θ) is defined in the transverse plane from -180 degrees to 180 degrees with 0 degrees at the x axis and positive Θ to the right side of the head. The elevation (α) is defined from a horizontal plane through the center of gravity (CG) of the head, 0 degrees, to the crown of the head at the z axis, 90 degrees. The elevation angle is described as the angle between the projected impact direction vector through the estimated head CG and a horizontal plane through the heads CG

(Crisco et al., 2004). Any impact above an elevation of 65° was considered a crown impact. The remaining four groups were based on azimuth; back (-45 degrees to 45 degrees), right side (45 degrees to 135 degrees), left side (-45 degrees to -135 degrees), and front (135 degrees to -135 degrees).

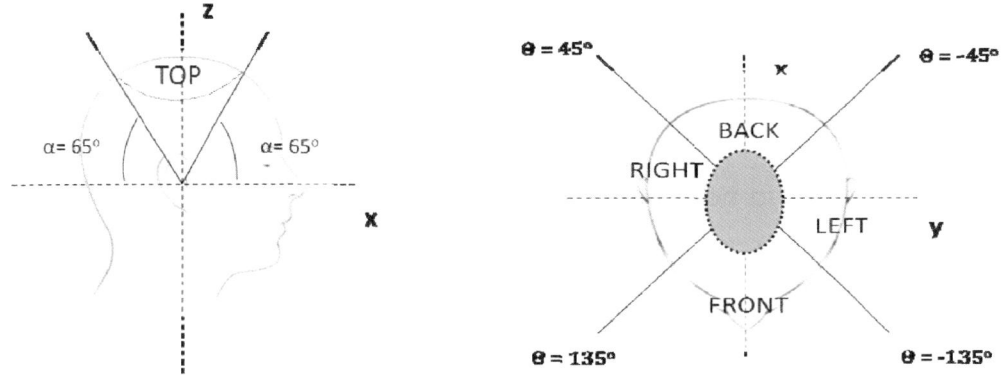

Figure 4.4: General impact locations

Cognitive Assessment - ImPACT

To effectively assess cognitive changes in the boxers, ImPACT© Version 5.0 was utilized to measure multiple aspects of cognitive functioning post-impact. For this study, the baseline test was obtained up to 24 hours prior to the bout. Post-impact tests were obtained immediately after and 24 hours after the bout has concluded. Each athlete was set up on a laptop computer with a mouse to insure ease and efficiency throughout the different modules. The laptop computers were set up in an area that best secluded the athletes from noise and distraction.

There are three different sections to the program that assist in the dynamic nature of the software. The first section is the subject profile and the health history questionnaire. The second section inquires about the athlete's current symptoms and conditions. And the final section is the neuropsychological test which includes six different modules that quantify how the athlete responds during the baseline and post-impact tests. The six different modules are: word discrimination, design memory, X's and O's, symbol matching, color match, and three letters.

The *word discrimination module* evaluates attentional processes, verbal recognition memory, and utilizes a word discrimination paradigm. This module provides a total percent correct score. The *design memory module* evaluates attentional processes, verbal recognition memory, and utilizes a design discrimination paradigm. The design memory module also provides a total percent correct score. The *X's and O's module* measures visual working memory as well as visual processing speed and consists of a visual memory paradigm with a distractor track. The distractor is a tool to measure the athlete's choice reaction time. Scores are provided for correct identification of the X's and O's, reaction time for the distractor task, and number of errors on the distractor task. The *symbol matching module* evaluates visual processing speed, learning and memory. This module provides an average reaction time score and a score for the memory condition. The *color matching module* represents a choice reaction time task and also measures impulse control and response inhibition. The color matching module provides a reaction time score and an error score. And finally, the *three letter module* measures the working memory and visual-motor response speed. This module yields a memory score, number of correctly identified letters, and a score for the average number of correctly clicked numbers per trial from the distractor test.

The scores that result from the modules during the post-impact tests are compared to the module results from the baseline test that was administered pre-impact. There are seven final composite scores that are calculated from the six modules: The *verbal memory* composite score is generated by performance on tests of word learning, word recognition memory and letter memory. This score is the average percent correct on the word discrimination module, the symbol match module, and the three letter module with an accompanying interference task. The *visual memory* composite is comprised of tests revealing shape learning and memory, visual working memory and visual associated memory. The visual memory score is calculated by taking the averages of the total percent correct score from the design memory module and total correct memory score from the X's and O's module. The *verbal* and *visual memory* composite scores represent the athlete's attention and memory capabilities. If there is a decrease in the scores, the athlete's ability to remember and/or remain attentive has been compromised. The *visual motor speed* is computed by taking the weighted averages of three tasks that are done as interference tasks for the memory paradigm. The following scores: total number correct divided by 4 during interference of the X's and O's module, and the average counted correctly multiplied by 3 from countdown phase of the three letter module comprise the score for the visual motor speed. The *reaction time* represents the average response time (in milliseconds) and is comprised of the average correct reaction time of the interference stage during the X's and O's module, average correct reaction time of the symbol match module divided by 3, and the average correct reaction time of the color match module. The *reaction time* and *visual motor speed* composite scores are demonstrative of the athlete's cognitive speed. An increase in the reaction time and a decrease in processing speed are evident of a decrease in the athlete's ability to recall new information in a timely manner. The *immediate memory score* is calculated by averaging the learning percent correct scores from the word memory and design memory modules. The immediate memory score provides information regarding the athlete's ability to immediately recall new information. The *delayed memory score* is determined by averaging the delayed memory percent scores from the word memory and design memory scores. The delayed memory score provides information regarding retention of newly learned information across the testing period. The final tabulated score is *working memory*. The following module scores are averaged to obtain the score for working memory: the X's and O's total correct (memory), the symbol match total correct (hidden) and the total sequence correct score from the three letters module. The working memory supplemental score is designed to provide information regarding the athlete's capacity to learn and retain information under conditions of interference.

Test Setup

Prior to the sparring session, each boxer completed baseline testing using the ImPACT© Version 5.0 cognitive software. Boxers were instructed to spar for 4-two minute rounds with an opponent of the same weight class and gender. Post-bout cognitive tests were obtained within 30 minutes and 24 hours following the sparring session. Each athlete performed the brief computerized test on a laptop computer with a mouse in a quiet area of the boxing facility. Post-bout physician assessments involved a basic evaluation of the boxer after the sparring session. Each athlete was assessed, by a ring-side physician when possible, for signs of MTBI or TBI using a standardized methodology employed by USA boxing.

Impact data from the headgear were post-processed by researchers at Simbex Inc. using an algorithm to calculate head acceleration, injury criterion, and impact location (Beckwith *et al.*, 2007). The scores that resulted from the modules during the post-bout tests were compared to the module results from the baseline test. From this comparison several scores were generated to assess the boxer's memory, attention, problem solving, and reaction time.

4.3 Statistical Analysis

The IBH and cognitive function data were analyzed using Statistical Package for Social Sciences (SPSS) version 16.0.2. An ANOVA was conducted when comparing the mean and peak values for the head acceleration and injury criterion between genders; however, violations of the normality assumption occurred and nonparametric tests (Mann-Whitney) were used to make the comparison. The comparison of the number of impacts sustained between genders was analyzed using a t-test. An Oneway ANOVA was used for the impact location data to determine the equality of the means without grouping by gender. For the cognitive data a Repeated Measures ANOVA was applied to analyze scores between and within gender groups. If a violation of the normality occurred, the nonparametric test Mann-Whitney Test for between group comparisons and Wilcoxon Signed Ranks Test for within group comparisons was utilized. For all tests with multiple comparisons, Bonferroni adjustments were made to decrease the number of Type I errors. A Pearson's correlation was used to compare the descriptive bout data (boxer's weight and number of impacts) and risk of injury parameters. In addition, a Pearson's correlation was conducted to compare the average values for the impact biomechanical data and cognitive test scores.

4.4 Results

Impact Boxing Headgear

Five participants withdrew from the study prior to the sparring session because cheek protectors were not an option on the instrumented headgear; therefore, the IBH data (Tables 4.1 and 4.2) included 55 participants with 1930 impacts. Twenty seven of the participants were males with 1128 impacts (42 impacts/boxer) and the remaining 28 participants were females with 802 impacts (29 impacts/boxer).

Table 4.1. Descriptive statistics for mean IBH impact data (‡ $p < 0.05$)

	Number of Impacts‡	HIC15	GSI	Translational Peak (g)	Rotational Peak (rad/s^2)
Male	42±27	43±100	66±148	30±21	2571±1852
Female	29±18	32±66	49±93	28±17	2533±1524

Table 4.2. Descriptive statistics for peak IBH impact data (‡ $p < 0.05$)

	Number of Impacts	HIC15‡	GSI‡	Translational Peak (g) ‡	Rotational Peak (rad/s^2) ‡
Male	104	1652	2292	191	17156
Female	83	1079	1487	184	13113

No significant difference was found for the mean head acceleration and injury criterion when comparing gender groups using the nonparametric Mann-Whitney test. The peak HIC, GSI, translational acceleration and rotational acceleration values were also compared by gender groups. Male boxers experienced a significantly higher peak translational acceleration ($p = 0.006$), HIC ($p = 0.005$), and GSI ($p = 0.005$) when compared to female boxers with an adjusted alpha level of $\alpha = 0.0125$. The peak rotational accelerations exhibited a mild level significance ($p = 0.013$). Additionally, a t-test was performed to compare the mean number of impacts between gender groups.

The male boxers had a significantly higher number of impacts (41.8 impacts/boxer) when compared to the female boxers (28.6 impacts/boxer) ($p = 0.04$) (Table 4.1).

To determine if a boxer's weight has any effect on the severity of impacts generated, a Pearson's correlation was used (Tables 4.3 and 4.4). All athletes sparred with a partner in the same weight class, therefore the weight of the boxer delivering the punches was assumed to be approximately the same as the boxer receiving the punches. For the male athletes the weight was found to have a weak negative linear relationship with the head accelerations (Table 4.3). A weak linear relationship was also found between the number of impacts and head accelerations and HIC. On the other hand, for female athletes a weak positive linear relation was found between weight and head acceleration (Table 4.4). Although these values are statistically significant, the linear relationships are weak.

Table 4.3. Correlation between weight and risk of injury parameters for male athletes (‡ $p < 0.05$ and ‡‡ $p < 0.01$)

	Number of Impacts	Weight	Translational Accel.	Rotational Accel.	HIC
Number of Impacts	1	0.091	-0.561‡‡	-0.565‡‡	-0.418‡
Weight	0.091	1	-0.473‡	-0.498‡	-0.349
Translational Accel.	-0.561‡‡	-0.473‡	1	0.968‡‡	0.910‡‡
Rotational Accel.	-0.565‡‡	-0.498‡	0.968‡‡	1	0.856‡‡
HIC	-0.418‡	-0.349	0.910‡‡	0.856‡‡	1

Table 4.4. Correlation between weight and risk of injury parameters for female athletes (‡ p < 0.05 and ‡‡ p < 0.01)

	Number of Impacts	Weight	Translational Accel.	Rotational Accel.	HIC
Number of Impacts	1	-0.015	-0.158	-0.187	0.018
Weight	-0.015	1	0.441‡	0.410‡	0.409‡
Translational Accel.	-0.158	0.441‡	1	0.955‡‡	0.840‡‡
Rotational Accel.	-0.187	0.410‡	0.955‡‡	1	0.728‡‡
HIC	0.018	0.409‡	0.840‡‡	0.728‡‡	1

Figures 4.5-4.7 illustrate the majority of the impacts sustained by the boxers were below the 25% probability threshold for brain injury established by Zhang *et al.* (2004). Combining the male and female data, 94.8% of the impacts where under the suggested translational acceleration threshold and 89.6% of the impacts where under the suggested rotational acceleration threshold. The percentage of impacts experienced by both genders that were under the MTBI threshold of 250, suggested by Pellman *et al.* (2003), was 97.8%.

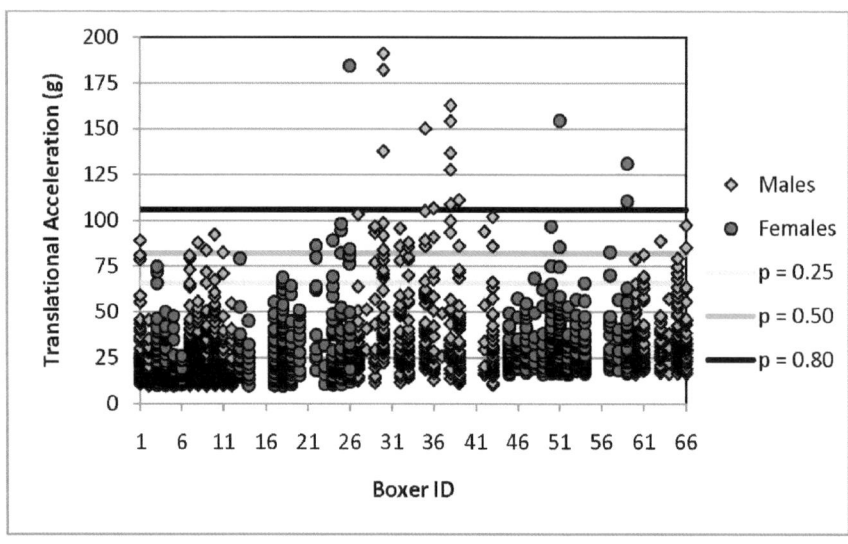

Figure 4.5: Male and female translational accelerations for each impact

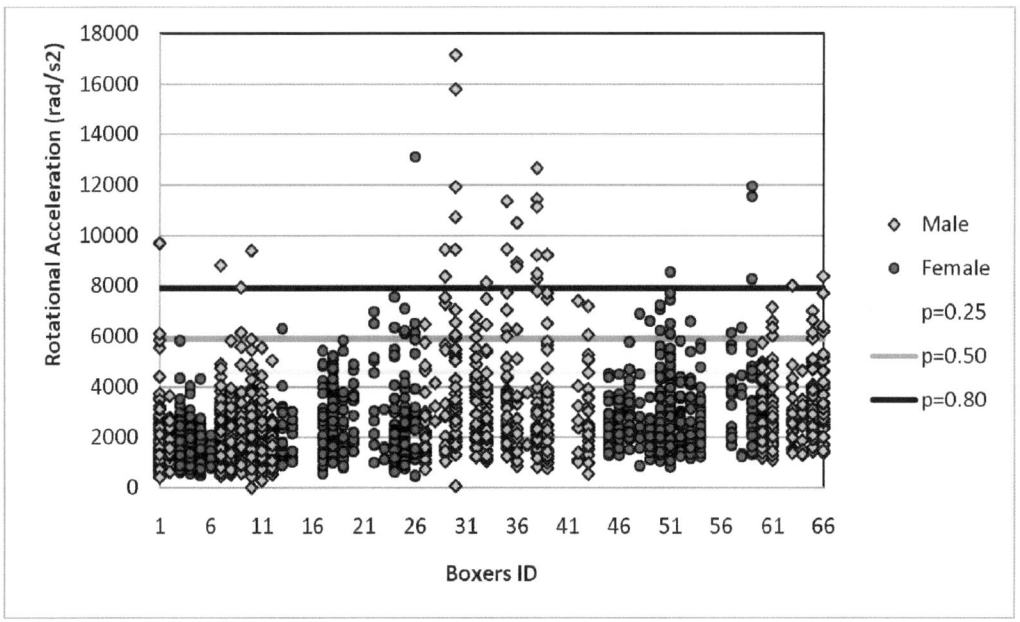

Figure 4.6: Male and female rotational acceleration for each impact

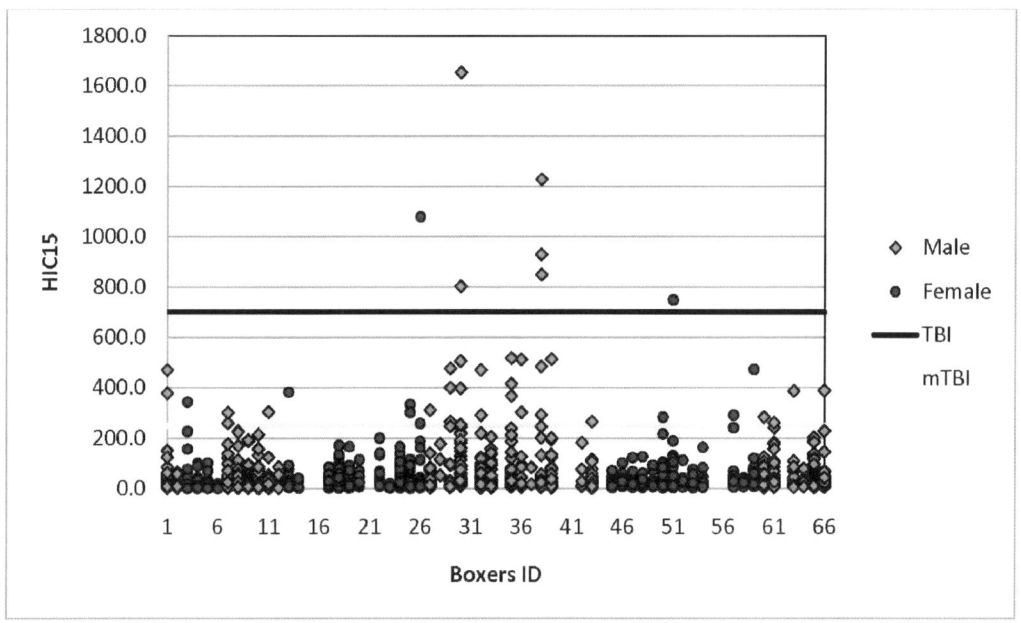

Figure 4.7: Male and female HIC scores for each impact

Figure 4.8 illustrates the total number of impacts that were sustained by all of the boxers grouped by location. An Oneway ANOVA was used to make the comparisons between the total number of impacts (n = 1930) to each region of the head. With an adjusted alpha value, α = 0.0125, the total number of impacts to the front region of the head (56%) was significantly higher when compared to the other locations (p < 0.001): left (17%), right (14%), back (11%), and top (2%). Although the male boxers experienced a higher number of impacts, the impact location trend was comparable for both genders.

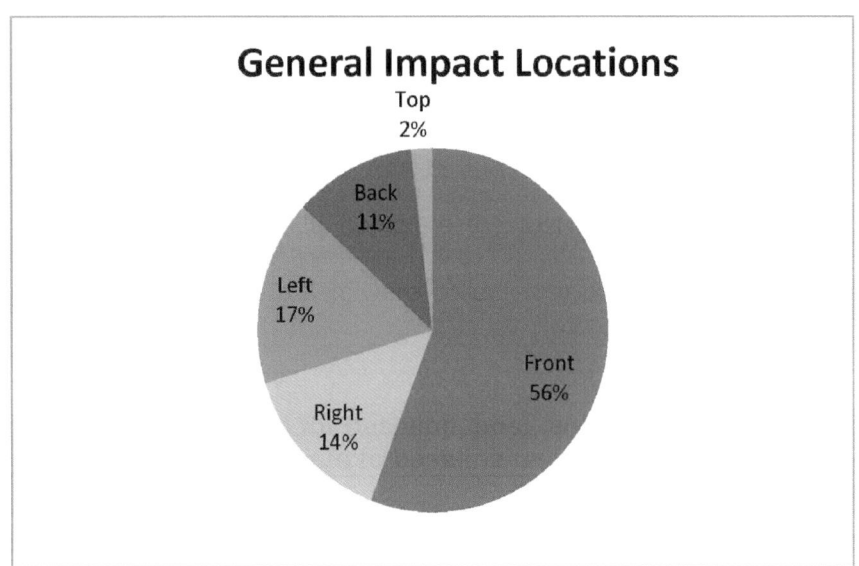

Figure 4.8: General locations for each impact sustained

The mean accelerations and HIC scores were compared by general impact location using the nonparametric Mann-Whitney test. No significant difference was observed between gender groups. Impacts to the front and top locations of the head were statistically significant when compared to the other locations (Table 4.5). Mean translational acceleration for the front was significantly lower compared to the back (p ≤ 0.01), right (p = 0.009), and left (p = 0.003) regions, mean rotational acceleration was significantly lower compared to the three regions (p ≤ 0.01) as well, and the mean HIC score was significantly lower compared to the back (p = 0.011) and left (p = 0.007) regions. The mean translational acceleration and mean HIC score for the top location were significantly lower when compared to the back, right, and left regions (p ≤ 0.01). Additionally, the mean rotational acceleration was significantly lower than the back (p = 0.012) and left (p = 0.013) regions in comparison to the top location. The values remain significant with an adjusted alpha value of α = 0.0167 due to repeated comparisons.

Table 4.5. General locations and corresponding mean accelerations and injury severity (‡ p<0.05, ‡*Mean score was not significant when comparing the front and top to the right values, but was significant when compared to the back and left values)

	Translational Acceleration (g's)	Rotational Acceleration (rad/s^2)	HIC
Front	27±18‡	2307±1587‡	33±81‡*
Right	31±19	2809±1705	43±78
Left	32±22	2898±1874	47±97
Top	20±14‡	2251±1410‡*	16±27‡
Back	34±25	3004±1982	52±116

Figure 4.9 depicts a graph of the rotational and translational accelerations for each impact. The impacts are labeled by the general location. The impacts with the highest rotational and translational accelerations were front impacts. The shaded box in the lower left corner of the graph illustrates the impacts that are below the 25% probability of brain damage established by Zhang et al. (2004).

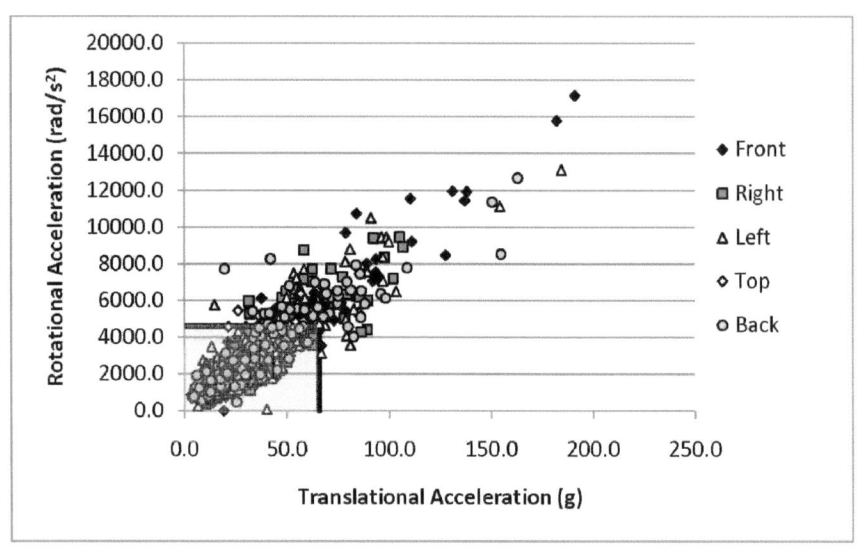

Figure 4.9: Rotational and translational accelerations of each impact based on general location

Neurocognitive assessment

Five athletes were unable to complete the testing series for various reasons; therefore, complete cognitive data sets were collected from 55 boxers, twenty six males and 29 females (Table 4.6).

Table 4.6: Mean ImPACT scores for baseline, post, and 24 hours post bout tests. (‡ $p < 0.05$ Comparison of post tests to baseline test)

	Baseline		Post		24 Hour Post	
	Male	Female	Male	Female	Male	Female
Verbal Memory	80±10	80±10	81±10	82±11	82±11	84±9
Visual Memory	68±13	65±13	70±13	61±14	69±14	69±13
Visual Motor Speed	33.7±8.8	32.8±8.1	34.9±8.4	37.4±7.6	35.3±9.3	37.0±7.9
Reaction Time	0.61±0.09	0.64±0.16	0.57±0.11	0.60±0.12	0.60±0.08	0.59±0.10
Immediate Memory	0.87±0.05	0.85±0.07	0.84±0.09	0.83±0.08	0.86±0.09	0.86±0.06
Delayed Memory	0.80±0.06	0.79±0.07	0.73±0.14‡	0.74±0.09‡	0.75±0.14	0.76±0.08
Working Memory	0.66±0.15	0.64±0.14	0.72±0.11	0.67±0.14	0.72±0.14	0.73±0.15

Both parametric and nonparametric tests were utilized when appropriate and proved that there was no significant difference when analyzing between gender groups.

However, a significant decrease was reported for the delayed memory post scores when analyzing the data using Repeated Measures ANOVA. A Pairwise Comparison of the three time points for delayed memory revealed significance between the baseline test and the post test for both males and females ($p \leq 0.01$) with an adjusted alpha value for multiple tests, $\alpha = 0.025$. The other scores either increased following the sparring session or did not significantly decrease when compared to the baseline tests. In addition, Pearson's correlations between the head accelerations, HIC, number of impacts, and cognitive scores were also investigated but the results were not clinically significant.

4.5 Discussion

The purpose of this study was to measure and analyze several biomechanical factors (translational acceleration, rotational acceleration, HIC, GSI, and impact location) during sparring sessions, in addition to collecting cognitive data. Amateur boxers volunteered for the study from various gyms, clubs and training camps. The IBH system was utilized to collect head impact data in the ring, while neurocognitive functions were assessed prior to sparring and at two time points following the sparring session.

The current research revealed the mean magnitude of the impacts, obtained by the IBH system, were lower than previously reported in the literature (Table 4.7). All the data yielded from previously published literature had been obtained through the use of impacting a surrogate by boxers performing a maximum impact. The setting of the current study involved collecting data during sparring sessions and therefore the levels of impacts observed may be lower than what would be recorded during competitive bouts. Further research should be conducted to determine whether the factor of competition would significantly increase the impacts experienced, and ultimately the cognitive function of the athletes. Although the sparring scenario provides the ability to have a more controlled study, competitive bouts would provide more realistic data. The majority of the impacts sustained in this study were sub-concussive and no concussions were noted in any of the participants following the sparring sessions. It is anticipated that more concussive events would be captured in a competition setting.

Table 4.7: Comparison of data found in literature for male boxers

	Trans. Accel. (g's)	Rot. Accel. (rad/s^2)	HIC
Current Study	30±21	2571±1852	43±100
Atha et al. (1985)	53	-	-
Walilko et al. (2005)	58±13	6343±1789	71±49
Stojsih et al. (2010)	49±23	5322±3010	54±52

Additionally, the general locations of each impact were determined by the IBH system. Research has indicated that acceleration, duration, and direction of the impact load may influence the outcome of an impact to the head (Versace, 1971; Ommaya and Gennarelli, 1974; Zhang et al., 2001; Kleiven, 2003; Pellman et al., 2003; Zhang et al., 2004; Delaney et al., 2006). Impacts in the lateral direction have been documented to result in brain injury more frequently (Zhang et al., 2001; Delaney et al., 2006). The current study revealed impacts to either side or back of the head exhibited, on average, significantly higher accelerations and HIC scores ($p < 0.05$). The impacts to the front region of the head produced significantly lower mean acceleration values which may be a result of specific training activities or preparation for the impact. Some athletes focus on building their cervical neck muscles to aid in the incidence or severity of concussion injury by absorbing the energy of the impact and minimize the movement of the head

(Cross and Serenelli, 2003) The frequency of the impacts to the front region of the head could be an additional explanation for the low head accelerations experienced by the athletes The number of impacts to the front region of the head represents over half of all the impacts sustained, indicating athletes may be more prepared for those impacts If the athletes are expecting impacts to the front of the head, preparation may be taken by activating muscles resulting in lower head accelerations experienced

While there is some data investigating the punch forces of male boxers (Atha *et al*, 1985, Smith *et al*, 2000, Walilko *et al*, 2005), the literature regarding female boxers is limited This study provides one of the first analyses of in-ring biomechanical data and cognitive function in female amateur boxers along with a comparison of the male and female data When analyzing the mean IBH impact data, many of the peak values exhibited a significant difference when comparing the male and female boxers In addition, the frequency of impacts sustained by the male boxers was significantly higher ($p < 0.05$) than the frequency sustained by the female boxers However, there were no significant differences in the mean translational and rotational accelerations, HIC, and GSI between genders (Table 4 1) On average the male boxers experienced more impacts, but the magnitude of the impacts for both genders was similar The cognitive function data proved that there was no difference between genders in their memory, attention, reaction time, and problem solving following the sparring sessions

Head accelerations and injury severity scores obtained from each impact during the sparring proved the majority of the impacts were below suggested injury thresholds (Zhang *et al*, 2004) The neurocognitive tests indicated that the athletes had difficulties retaining information during the post-sparring test as indicated in a significant decrease in the delayed memory scores. This finding indicates that immediately after a boxer spars, retention of new information is compromised. Twenty four hours after the bout, the delayed memory score still was lower than the baseline, however, it was not significant. The present results compliment the results yielded in a study by Heilbronner *et al* where neuropsychological tests were administered to 23 amateur boxers (Heilbronner *et al*, 1991). Comparison of test scores before and after a single sparring session showed a deficit in verbal memory and incidental (delayed) memory in the amateur boxers.

In contrast, other studies have found no relationship between boxing and cognitive dysfunction. Moriarity *et al* followed 82 amateur boxers in a 7-day tournament and assessed their cognitive functioning following the bouts (Moriarity *et al*, 2004). It was found that the amateur boxers showed no evidence of cognitive dysfunction in the immediate post bout period. In a 9 year prospective study of amateur boxers, Porter found that the boxers exhibited no evidence of neuropsychological deterioration (Porter, 2003). Other studies also support this conclusion (Brooks *et al*, 1987, Butler, 1994). Although Butler (1994) found no sign of neuropsychological dysfunction, it was suggested that a long amateur career might reduce fine motor movements. More extensive data is needed over a longer time line to determine the potential effects of repetitive concussive and sub-concussive head impacts in amateur boxers.

There are several advantages and disadvantages when implementing a computerized neuropsychological test system. Such tools are easy to use, especially with large groups, and allow for a comparison between baseline test results. However, when testing an athlete for the first time there is a possibility that the baseline test could be invalid. This may occur if the athlete does not concentrate, fails to carefully read through directions, or is surrounded by distractions. If possible, to minimize these problems, prior to the baseline explain what the athletes should expect from the test and be sure the environment is free of distractions. Also, with repetitive test taking, there may be a learning effect that could confound the results. Therefore, such tests should not be the sole predictor of concussion assessment. The clinical evaluation and other tools should be included and the results of all tests should be evaluated together.

This study represents the first in-ring collection of impact data for both male and female amateur boxers. These findings are an important contribution to both impact biomechanics and cognitive impairment research. Further efforts will enhance the body of knowledge related to sports-related brain injury. It is critical to determine thresholds of injury so that protective measures, including headgear and gloves, may be properly evaluated.

CHAPTER 5 – BIOMECHANICS OF COMPETITION

5.1 Introduction

Amateur boxing has evolved as a way to make boxing a safer sport for a broad range of athletes. During competitions, amateur bouts are limited to three or four – two minute rounds, scoring is based on the number of clean blows landed, and athletes are required to wear protective headgear and mouth guards to reduce the risk of injuries. In order to score points one must impact the head or torso of their opponent. Other locations are off limits or do not count. To ensure a win, knock outs are usually desired, consequently the head is the main target.

According to a study conducted by Porter and O'Brien (1996), approximately half of the injuries sustained by amateur boxers during competition were concussions. Zazryn et al. (2006) discovered 25% of injuries sustained to the head of an amateur boxer were concussions during competition. Although, the majority of head injuries occur during competitions, this is the first study to assess the severity of impacts to the head during a competitive bout.

Stojsih et al. (2008) was the first to use a wireless telemetry system in the ring and compared the acceleration levels of male and female amateur boxers. Boxers were asked to wear an instrumented headgear developed by Simbex Inc. (Lebanon, NH). Real-time head acceleration data and head injury criterion where collected for each impact during the 4-two minute round sessions. In addition to collecting biomechanical data, cognitive data were collected before and twice after the session. This study found that there was no significant difference between the male and female head acceleration data and suggested that female amateur boxers were not at a greater risk for head injury when compared to male data. Since the literature has found that the majority of head injuries occur during competition and not training, both biomechanical and cognitive data should be collected during a competitive bout.

Therefore the goal of this study was to collect data in the ring during competition. The Instrumented Boxing Headgear (IBH) developed by Simbex was used for this study (Stojsih et al., 2008). The head acceleration, HIC, and GSI were recorded for each impact. In addition, cognitive function was assessed before and after the bouts.

5.2 Methods

Sample Population

Amateur boxers were recruited during registration periods at the 2008 and 2009 Ringside World Championships in Kansas City, Missouri. Thirty six amateur boxers (34 male and 2 female) participated in August 2008 and fourteen amateur boxers (13 male and 1 female) participated in August 2009. All athletes were over 18 years of age. Approval was garnered from the Wayne State University Human Investigation Committee prior to testing with all subjects consenting to participate prior to testing.

IBH System

In an effort to collect in-ring head accelerations, the use of the Instrumented Boxing Headgear (IBH) system was developed by Simbex Inc. (Lebanon, NH). The IBH system is designed after the Head Impact Telemetry System (HITS) which Simbex developed for use in football helmets. The only difference between the two systems is the amount of single-axis accelerometers. Twelve accelerometers are placed in an array in between the head-side leather and padding of the headgear's backside and rear pads for the IBH system. Placement of the accelerometers was based on the need to minimize the probability of direct contact from an impact. The battery pack and radio were inserted into the rear panel of the headgear between the outside leather and foam pad. The accelerometers, battery, and data acquisition and radio hardware increased headgear weight by only 4 oz (Beckwith *et al.*, 2007). Each headgear is considered one unit and the data from that unit were transferred via radio frequency to a wireless receiver and laptop computer system. For each impact the time, linear acceleration, rotational acceleration, GSI, and HIC are downloaded to the on-board memory.

Cognitive Assessment - SAC

For the cognitive assessment, it was determined that the Standardized Assessment of Concussion (SAC) would be most appropriate. The ImPACT cognitive test utilized when collecting sparring data had its limitations, including the amount of time needed for each test. The SAC (McCrea *et al.*, 1997), distributed by CSMi Medical Solutions (Stoughton, MA), is a method used to supplement on-field assessment of athletes suspected of MTBI. The system was developed to provide a clinician with a standardized, objective measure for assessing the immediate neurocognitive and neurological effects of concussion. There are four major domains of function that were assessed during training: orientation, immediate memory, concentration, and delayed recall. The orientation section is used to assess a subject's awareness of current situation and surroundings. The subject is asked to provide the day of the week, month, date, year and time of day within one hour. The Immediate Memory section is used to assess a subject's ability to encode information and learn new information. A 5-word list is used to measure immediate memory, as the subject is read the list and required to repeat back as many as he or she can remember, and the procedure is repeated for three trials. The concentration portion is used to evaluate the subject for deficits in attention, concentration, information processing and working memory. There are two parts to the concentration section, reciting digits backwards (3 to 6 series of numbers) and the months of the year in reverse order. The final section, delayed recall is utilized to assess the subject's ability to retain newly-learned information over time. Recall of the 5-word list used for the Immediate Memory section is ascertained without forewarning or recall cues.

From the four sections of the test a total score is computed in order to derive a composite index of the subjects overall level of impairment following concussion. The maximum total score on the SAC is 30 points. The SAC requires approximately 5-7 minutes administering in most cases and is completed on an individual basis. The test has three different forms (A, B, and C) that can be used. The three SAC forms have different lists of words and digits to insure variation and minimize the practice effect.

Test Setup

After participants consented, each subject was escorted to an area where the ringside physician administer the baseline SAC. Once each subject had finished the baseline test, they were fitted with the appropriate instrumented headgear. The headgear ranged from small, medium, or large and were available with or without check pads. Boxers were asked to wear the headgear during their bout. Each bout was either 2 or 3-two minute rounds, depending on whether the bout was stopped early. Data were only collected during one bout for each participant. The IBH recorded head acceleration, injury criterion, duration, location, and time for each impact. Following the bout, the athletes were then administered a second SAC exam. Form A was used for the baseline and Form B was used for the post-bout assessment (Appendix C). An alternate form was used for the follow up test to minimize practice effect in order to track potential injury. The surrounding environment was similar for both tests to help prevent any additional extraneous factors.

5.3 Statistical Analysis

The overall SAC scores and sub-scores were analyzed using the PASW (Predictive Analytics Software, formerly SPSS) Statistics 18 (IBM Inc., Chicago IL). A non parametric test was utilized for the analysis. The 2-tailed exact significance is reported. The total number of impacts for each athlete was compared for the different regions of the head using a One-Way ANOVA. Pearson's correlation was used to compare descriptive bout data (boxer weight and number of impacts) and risk of injury parameters. Additionally, Pearson's correlation was used to determine if there is a linear relationship between the cognitive test scores and biomechanical data collected from the headgear.

5.4 Results

Although data were collected from 50 boxers, data from only fifteen males were suitable for inclusion. Initially the same SAC forms were used for baseline and post bout cognitive testing. It was decided to minimize the practice effect, therefore, data from participants tested with two different SAC forms were only included in the analysis. In addition, during the 2009 data collection, one of the instrumented headgear experienced a short in the player unit resulting in erroneous data.

Impact Boxing Headgear

The IBH data included 15 male participants with 805 impacts. All of the participants were male amateur boxers with an average of 54 impacts per boxer per bout. Table 5.1 illustrates the average and peak data recorded by the Impact Boxing Headgear. To determine if there was a linear relationship between data collected using the IBH (head acceleration and injury criterion) compared to the weight of the boxer and the number of impacts sustained, a Pearson's correlation was conducted. The results indicated that there was no relationship between the variables. This could, however, be an effect of the small sample size.

Table 5.1: Mean and peak IBH impact data

	Number of Impacts	HIC15	Translational Peak (g)	Rotational Peak (rad/s^2)
Mean	54±27	44±100	29±21	2240±1592
Maximum	95	981	178	10163

Figures 5.1-5.3 illustrate that the majority of the impacts were below thresholds designated by Zhang *et al.* (2004). Combining all of the impacts, 94% were below the 25% probability of a mild head injury when comparing translational acceleration to the suggested thresholds. For the rotational head acceleration, 91% of the impacts were below the suggested threshold (Zhang *et al.*, 2004). The threshold for a concussion based on HIC score is suggested at 250 (Pellman *et al.*, 2003). The percentage of impacts sustained by athletes that were under 250 was 96%. The majority of the impacts recorded in this study were sub-concussive.

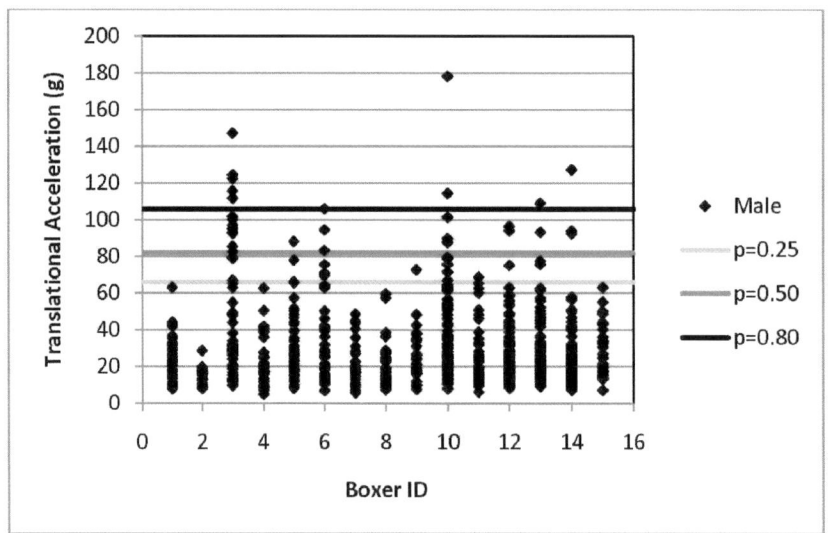

Figure 5.1: Translational head accelerations for each impact

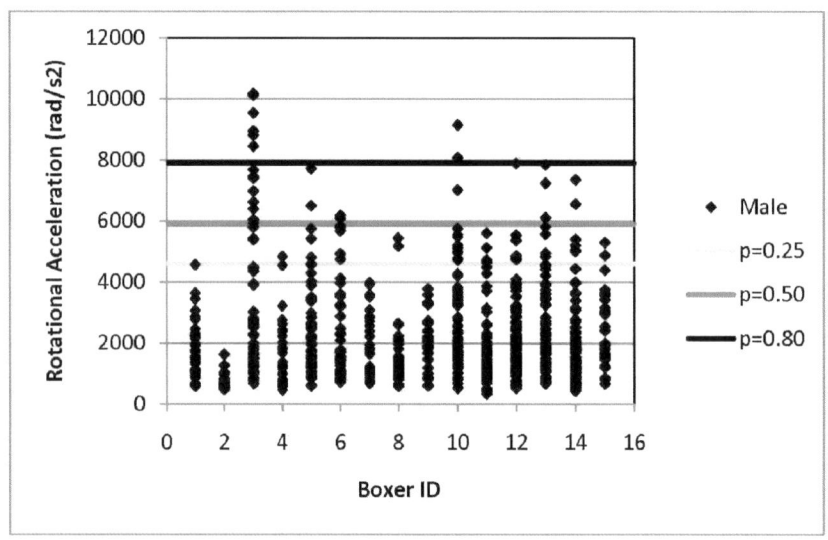

Figure 5.2: Rotational head accelerations for each impact

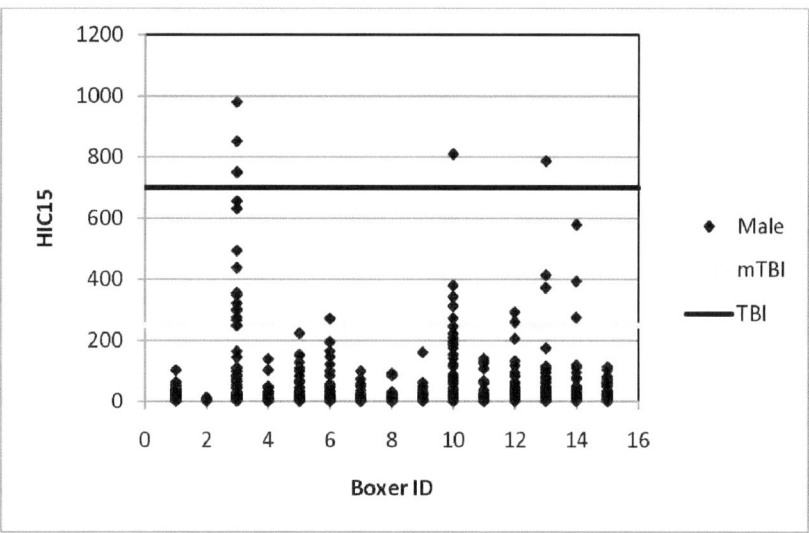

Figure 5.3: HIC scores for each impact

Figure 5.4 illustrates the total number of impacts that were sustained by all of the boxers grouped by location. A Repeated Measure ANOVA was used to make the comparisons between the total number of impacts to each region of the head. The total number of impacts to the front region of the head (34%) was significantly higher when compared to the other locations ($p < 0.01$): right (21%), left (18%), and top (3%). The number of impacts to the front of the head was not significantly different than the number to the back of the head ($p = 0.192$). While it is considered a foul to punch an opponent in the back of the head during a competition, the high number of impacts to the back of the head may be a result of how the impact locations are defined in the IBH system. If the impact is near 45° azimuth on the right side or -45° on the left side it may register as an impact to the rear of the head (Figure 4.4).

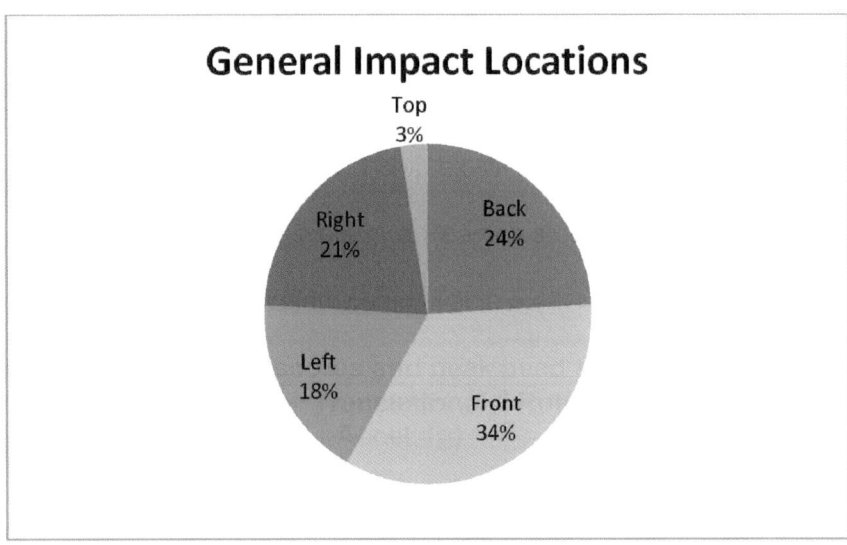

Figure 5.4: General locations for each impact sustained.

The mean accelerations and HIC scores were compared by general impact location using the nonparametric Mann-Whitney test. There was no statistical significance when comparing the head accelerations and injury criterion by location of impact (Table 5.2). The values collected from the impacts to the top region of the head are visibly larger when compared to the other regions. This may be a result of such a small number of impacts occurring in that region (3%).

Table 5.2. General locations and corresponding mean accelerations and injury severity (‡ $p<0.05$)

	Translational Acceleration (g's)	Rotational Acceleration (rad/s^2)	HIC
Front	28±18	2101±1547	35±79
Right	32±26	2376±1686	54±119
Left	29±20	2281±1525	39±85
Top	39±37	3044±2962	129±221
Back	29±20	2200±1379	40±92

SAC

Figure 5.5 illustrates the overall baseline and post-bout SAC scores for all 15 athletes. Twelve athletes received lower scores following the bout; the remaining 3 scored the same or higher following the bout. On average, the amateur boxers dropped 2.1±2.2 from baseline immediately following the bout.

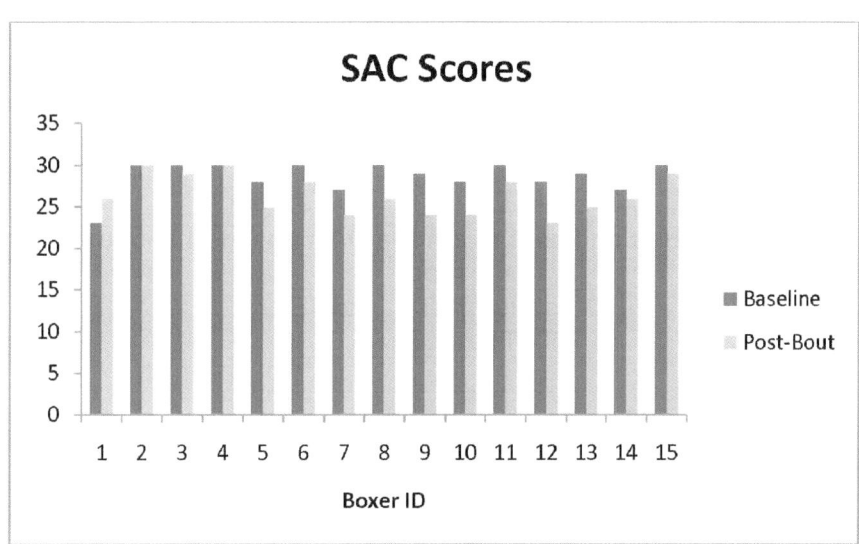

Figure 5.5: Overall Baseline and Post bout SAC scores

Table 5.3: Mean sub-scores and overall SAC scores. (‡ $p < 0.05$ Comparison of post tests to baseline test)

	Baseline	Post-bout	Difference ($T_2 - T_1$)
Orientation	5.0±0	4.9±0.3	-0.1±0.3
Immediate Memory	14.7±0.9	14.5±0.9	-0.2±0.9
Concentration	4.4±0.9	3.6±1.2‡	-0.8±1.2
Delay Recall	4.5±0.8	3.5±1.1‡	-1.1±1.3
Total Score	28.6±1.9	26.5±2.4‡	-2.1±2.2

Table 5.3 compares the baseline and post bout sub-scores for each athlete. The Wilcoxon Signed Ranks non-parametric test was used to compare the baseline and

post-bout SAC scores. The test revealed a significant difference between the concentration (p = 0.031) and delayed recall (p = 0.008) subtests and the total scores (p = 0.005). To determine if a linear relationship exists between the change in SAC scores and the data collected by the IBH system, a Pearson's correlation was conducted. The statistical test revealed no linear relationship (Table 5.4).

Table 5.4: Cognitive scores and peak head acceleration comparison

Boxer ID	Difference Score (T_2-T_1)	Translational Accel. (g)	Rotational Accel. (rad/s^2)	Number of Impacts
1	+3	63	4568	39
2	0	29	1623	16
3	-1	147	10163	55
4	0	63	4830	28
5	-3	88	7721	55
6	-2	106	6176	41
7	-3	48	3977	31
8	-4	59	5436	48
9	-5	73	3781	31
10	-4	178	9147	85
11	-2	69	5600	66
12	-5	96	7888	92
13	-4	109	7844	95
14	-1	127	7356	94
15	-1	63	5286	29

5.5 Discussion

Injuries in boxing, during both training and competition, have been well documented in the literature. The mechanism by which the injuries are caused, on the other hand, have yet to be established. This study collected in-ring head accelerations and injury criterion for each impact a given boxer experienced throughout the duration of one bout. In addition, neurocognitive data was collected before and after the bout.

One other study collected in-ring head acceleration data from amateur boxers using the IBH system (Stojsih *et al.*, 2008). Stojsih *et al.* (2008) collected biomechanical and cognitive data during sparring sessions. It is expected that the head accelerations generated during a competition would be higher than those generated during training. However, when comparing the two studies using the non parametric Mann-Whitney test the results were not significantly different ($p > 0.05$). The mean translational head acceleration generated during sparring for male amateur boxers was 30 ± 21 g and during competition was 29 ± 21 g. The mean rotational head acceleration generated during sparring was 2571 ± 1852 rad/s^2 and 2240 ± 1592 rad/s^2 from competition. Both the current study and Stojsih *et al.* (2008) found similar results when comparing the IBH data to injury thresholds. The majority of the impacts were below head acceleration thresholds suggested by Zhang *et al.* (2004). However, a study by Funk *et al.* suggested thresholds that are much higher for causing an MTBI (Funk *et al.*, 2007).

As a routine part to all competitions, boxers are given an exam administered by a ringside physician before and after their bout. A detailed physical exam is performed initially to determine whether the athlete is fit to box. Orientation, level of consciousness, and balance is tested at this time as well. Immediately after the athletes exit the ring a brief exam assessing the athletes' mental status, head, neck, or extremity injuries is given. If a boxer is knocked unconscious a more detailed and injury specific exam is administered. These examinations are important for identifying potentially life threatening conditions, but they are not adequately sensitive for detecting mild cognitive defects (Heilbronner *et al.*, 2009). An appropriate ringside neurological exam would include tests for orientation, attention, and the athlete's ability to learn new information and retain the information. The SAC is one example of a brief test that will evaluate the boxer's mental status and determine if there are signs of retrograde or post-traumatic amnesia. The SAC neurological exam that was given during this study was administered in addition to the ringside physicians' exam. The SAC is intended as a supplement to other methods of concussion assessment. According to the mandatory exam given by the physicians, the athletes in this study did not exhibit a concerning number of signs/symptoms to warrant further examination or withdrawal from the contact sport.

Previously published studies have been conducted utilizing the SAC exam to help identify mild head injuries on the sidelines (McCrea et al., 1997; McCrea et al., 1998; McCrea, 2001). One study evaluated 63 high school and collegiate football players that experienced a concussion (according to AAN guidelines) and compared cognitive data with 55 uninjured participants (McCrea, 2001). According to McCrea et al. (2001), injured subjects perform significantly below the pre-season baseline SAC total score (T_1 = 27.14±1.81, T_2 = 22.46±3.61) immediately after being injured, while uninjured participants did not (T_1 = 26.24±2.12, T_2 = 26.87±2.05). In addition, injured participants scored significantly below the pre-season baseline on the Orientation, Immediate Memory, Concentration, and Delayed Recall directly following injury. Ninety-five percent of the injured subjects demonstrated a drop of at least 1 point immediately after concussion, while only 24% of uninjured control experienced this drop (McCrea, 2001). A drop of 1 point or more from the baseline score was found to have a 95% sensitivity and 76% specific in identifying injured and uninjured participants correctly (McCrea, 2001).

According to the data collected during this study there was an average drop in the total score of the SAC of -2.5±2.6. Eighty percent of the participants demonstrated a drop of at least 1 point following the bout (Table 5.5). Two participants exhibited a decrease in the total score of more than 4 points. On average, following the bout, the largest decrease in points occurred during the Concentration and Delayed Recall sections of the SAC. Based on the results from this study, a test that is more sensitive (such as the SAC) should be used when evaluating the cognitive function of a boxer following a bout. Potential mild head injuries might be missed which could also increase the risk of a more severe head injury occurring if an athlete enters the ring with an undetected mild head injury.

Table 5.5: Differences between SAC scores at baseline and immediately following bout

Boxer ID	Difference Score (T_2-T_1)
1	+3
2	0
3	-1
4	0
5	-3
6	-2
7	-3
8	-4
9	-5
10	-4
11	-2
12	-5
13	-4
14	-1
15	-1

Future directions for this research should include recruiting more participants. The sample size for this study is fairly small and should be expanded to female participants as well. Relationships between the biomechanical and cognitive data could be determined with additional participants. Furthermore, collecting cognitive data 24 hours after the bout could provide insight into the recovery period of a concussion.

Although most of the impacts were sub-concussive and none of the participants were diagnosed with a concussion (based on AAN guidelines), this study was the first to collect real time data during a competition and these data illustrate the head accelerations and cognitive functioning of a boxer during one competitive bout

CHAPTER 6 – CONCLUSIONS AND FUTURE RECOMMENDATIONS

6.1 Conclusions

The origin of boxing, also known as the sweet science, dates back to ancient Greece and Rome where athletes wore leather straps wrapped around their fists and matches ended with serious injuries and sometimes even death. Today, the sport of boxing is less chaotic. Weight divisions, round limits, and referees are standard in modern competitions. As the sport continued to evolve, participants in Olympic and amateur boxing increased during the 20th century. Additionally, in the past two decades the popularity of the sport with females had increased. This was mainly a result of the USA boxing ban on females participating in the sport being lifted in 1993.

Boxing has been the focus of numerous studies published in peer reviewed journals. Researchers have investigated injuries, punch force, and overall biomechanics of Olympic-level, amateur, and professional boxers. However all of these studies have been carried out in the laboratory. The research currently presented was collected from amateur boxers in the laboratory and in the field. Punch force, cognitive functioning, and biomechanical data were collected to help understand the force exerted by different punches to the head and how the head responds for both male and female boxers over the age of 18 years. These are important concerns for injury prevention and protective equipment standards.

Male and female biomechanical data were collected during the punch force laboratory study and sparring sessions. The mean results from the punch force study yielded higher punch force, head acceleration, injury criterion, and hand velocity generated by male boxers. A significant difference was found when comparing the data generated by the three different punches for the male boxers. This difference was not present for the female boxers. When analyzing the sparring data results no significant difference between mean head acceleration and injury criterion scores were noted when comparing genders. However, the male boxers did experience significantly higher peak head accelerations and peak injury criterion scores when compared to the females. A significant difference also occurred between the mean number of impacts sustained during the 4-two minute rounds sparring sessions. Even though, on average, males and females are exposed to impacts of similar severity, male boxers sustain a significantly higher number of impacts during a sparring session. Unfortunately, female data was not obtained in the competitive setting and such gender comparisons could not be made. One common finding in all data collection settings was that the majority of impacts, for both males and females, were below suggested head injury thresholds by Zhang et al. (2004) and Pellman et al. (2003). An overwhelming majority of impacts that a boxer sustains, in both training and competition, are sub-concussive.

The purpose of sparring in the sport of boxing is to train for a competitive match without striking one's partner with maximum effort to avoid injury. Since these sessions are less intense compared to a competitive match one would assume fewer impacts would occur. However, based on the current research presented, the average number of impacts sustained by male boxers during a sparring session was slightly lower than the number sustained during a competition but the results were not statistically significant. Also, one would expect the head accelerations generated during sparring to be significantly lower when compared to impacts from competitions. During the current research this hypothesis was found not to be true. The head accelerations generated during a competition for male athletes were not significantly different than those generated during a sparring session.

The diagnosis and management of a concussion is one of the most complex challenges a ringside physician faces. Identifying a head injury is easier when there is a loss of consciousness; however, more than 90% of concussions fall into a milder category where there is no loss of consciousness but rather a brief period where alertness is lost (Cantu, 1996). Recognizing all concussions becomes very important when dealing with athletes that are exposed to direct head impacts often. Two different cognitive tests were utilized during this research. Both tests were used as a tool to identify subtle signs/symptoms of a mild head injury. The first exam, the ImPACT software, was utilized when collecting data from male and female amateur boxers before, immediately after, and 24 hours after a sparring session. The exam took approximately 30 minutes for the athletes to complete each time. The results of this test indicated a significant decrease in delayed memory immediately after the sparring session. This was the result for both genders and no significant difference was exhibited between genders. While this exam seemed more exact it was very time consuming and a few subjects were removed because they did not complete the last test. When collecting data during competitions a shorter cognitive test was utilized. The SAC exam is specifically for sideline identification of head injury. However, this exam should be used with another traditional form of cognitive assessment. During this study, ringside physicians administered a detailed exam before and after the bouts. The participants in this study seemed to exhibit an overall decrease of approximately 2 points. Although there was no indication of head injury during the ringside physician's exam, the SAC indicated at least 2 of the participants could have experienced an undetected mild head injury.

6.2 Future Recommendations

One of the major challenges of this study was subject recruitment. It was extremely difficult to recruit female boxers. Although boxing is increasing in popularity with females, it is still a male dominated sport. It was difficult to find females of the same weight class to spar one another and the number of females that attended the annual competition was minimal. Female competition data are needed to perform gender comparisons and to compare the female sparring data to competition data. Recruitment will continue at the annual Ringside competition and potentially other competitions to obtain more female specific data.

An additional population that could be analyzed would be participants under the age of 18. Boxing is a very popular sport with children especially in urban areas. The sport teaches children discipline, self-defense, and agility. And for some youths, the contact sport provides them with a structured and purpose oriented alternative to the streets. Collecting youth specific data would be beneficial when evaluating the standards since these data have yet to be published in the literature. However, recruiting youth participants may prove to be difficult since an assent form is needed from the parents in addition to consent from the child. Parents are not always present at competitions and a coach is not permitted to give the assent.

Collecting data from boxers that become concussed in the ring would be beneficial in determining injury thresholds and in evaluating and creating new equipment standards. This will also be a difficult population to obtain. From the literature, the majority of head injuries occur during competition bouts, therefore, more data must be collected during competitions

APPENDIX A – HIC Approvals

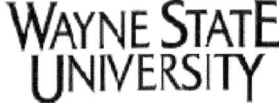

HUMAN INVESTIGATION COMMITTEE
St. Antoine Boulevard - LHC-6G
Detroit Michigan 48201
Phone: (313) 577-1628
FAX: (313) 993-7122
http://hic.wayne.edu

NOTICE OF FULL BOARD APPROVAL

To:	Marianne Wilhem Biomechanics Center Bioengineering Bldg.
From:	Virgiria Delaney-Black, M.D., MPH *M. Simon for* -MIA- Chairperson, Medical/Pediatric Institutional Review Board (MP4)
Date:	October 06, 2005
RE:	Protocol #: 0509002891 Protocol Title: Assessment of MTBI in Female Boxers Sponsor: 069247 Reference #1: 093405MP4F Reference #2:
Expiration Date:	September 21, 2006

The above-referenced Protocol and following information (if applicable) were **APPROVED** following Full Board Review by the Wayne State University Institutional Review Board (MP4) for the period of 10/06/2005 through 09/21/2006.

o Informed Consent Form (revised 10/4/05).

This approval does not replace any departmental or other approvals that may be required.

Federal regulations require that all research be reviewed at least annually. **It is the Principal Investigator's responsibility to obtain review and continued approval before the expiration date.** You may **not** continue any research activity beyond the expiration date without HIC approval.

- If you wish to have your protocol approved for continuation, please submit a completed Continuation Form** at least <u>six weeks</u> before the expiration date. It may take up to six weeks from the time of submission to the time of approval to process your continuation request.
- **Failure to receive approval for continuation before the expiration date will result in the automatic suspension of the approval of this protocol on the expiration date. Information collected following suspension is unapproved research and can <u>never</u> be reported or published as research data.**
- If you do not wish continued approval, please submit a completed Closure Form** when the study is terminated.
- All changes or amendments to your protocol or consent form require review and approval by the Human Investigation Committee (HIC) **BEFORE** implementation.
- You are also required to submit a written description of any adverse reactions or unexpected events on the appropriate form (Adverse Reaction and Unexpected Event Form*) within the specified time frame.

*Based on the Expedited Review List, revised November 1998

**Current version of the appropriate form(s) must be used (available on the HIC website).

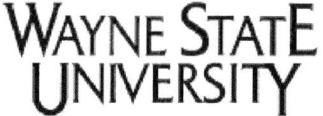

HUMAN INVESTIGATION COMMITTEE
101 East Alexandrine Building
Detroit Michigan 48201
Phone: (313) 577-1628
FAX: (313) 993-7122
http://hic.wayne.edu

NOTICE OF EXPEDITED AMENDMENT APPROVAL

To: Cynthia Bir
Biomechanics Center
818 Hancock, Bioengineering Ctr

From: Francis LeVeque, D.D.S.
Chairman, Human Investigation Committee

Date: January 26, 2007

RE: HIC#: 093405MP4F
Protocol Title: Assessment of MTBI in Female Boxers
Sponsor: NATIONAL OPERATING COMMITTEE ON STANDARDS FOR ATHL EQUIP.
Coeus #: 0509002891

Expiration Date: September 27, 2007

The above-referenced protocol amendment, as itemized below, was reviewed by the Chairman/designee of the Human Investigation Committee *for* the Wayne State University Institutional Review Board (MP4), and is **APPROVED** effective immediately.

- Addition of Sarah Stojsih as a co-investigator.
- Flyer and Consent Form (revised 1/25/07) - Both forms modifed to remove the blood draw procedure wording.
- Protocol - Modification of data collection methods to remove the blood draw.

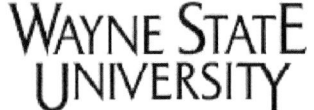
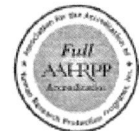

HUMAN INVESTIGATION COMMITTEE
101 East Alexandrine Building
Detroit, Michigan 48201
Phone: (313) 577-1628
FAX: (313) 993-7122
http://hic.wayne.edu

NOTICE OF EXPEDITED AMENDMENT APPROVAL

To: Cynthia Bir
Biomedical Engineering
818 Hancock, Bioengineering Ctr

From: Manuel Tancer, M.D.
Interim Chairman, Human Investigation Committee

Date: June 24, 2008

RE: HIC#: 093405MP4F
Protocol Title: Assessment of MTBI in Female Boxers
Sponsor: NATIONAL OPERATING COMMITTEE ON STANDARDS FOR ATHL EQUIP.
Coeus #: 0509002891

Expiration Date: August 22, 2008

The above-referenced protocol amendment, as itemized below, was reviewed by the Chairman/designee of the Human Investigation Committee *for* the Wayne State University Institutional Review Board (MP4), and is **APPROVED** effective immediately.

- Receipt of a revised flyer to ask for the participation of boxers that will be attending the competition
- Receipt of a revised narrative summary containing revised enrollment critria changes (Ringside Boxing Competition - Kansas City, Kansas) and revised data collection methods (revised concussion software administered by a physician)
- Receipt of a revised consent form (dated 06/09/2008) based on revised study procedures and enrollment criteria submitted

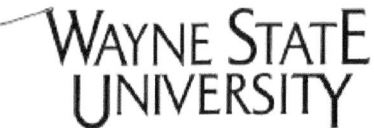
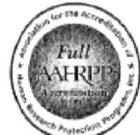

HUMAN INVESTIGATION COMMITTEE
101 East Alexandrine Building
Detroit, Michigan 48201
Phone: (313) 577-1628
FAX: (313) 993-7122
http://hic.wayne.edu

NOTICE OF FULL BOARD CONTINUATION APPROVAL

To: Cynthia Bir
Biomedical Engineering
818 Hancock, Bioengineering Ctr

From: Virginia Delaney-Black, M.D., M.P.H.
Chairperson, Medical/Pediatric Institutional Review Board (MP4)

Date: September 24, 2009

RE: HIC #: 093405MP4F
Protocol Title: Assessment of MTBI in Amateur Boxers
Sponsor: ° Biomedical Engineering
Protocol #: 0509002891

Expiration Date: September 23, 2010

Risk Level / Category: Adult: Research involving greater than minimal risk, presenting no prospect of direct benefit, but likely to yield generalizable knowledge about the participant's condition

Continuation for the above-referenced protocol and items listed below (if applicable) were **APPROVED** following Full Board review by the Wayne State University Institutional Review Board (MP4) for the period of 09/24/2009 through 09/23/2010. This approval does not replace any departmental or other approvals that may be required.

- Research Informed Consent (revision dated 7/27/09)
- Study Flyer

° Federal regulations require that all research be reviewed at least annually. You *may* receive a *"Continuation Renewal Reminder"* approximately two months prior to the expiration date; however, it is the Principal Investigator's responsibility to obtain review and continued approval *before* the expiration date. Data collected during a period of lapsed approval is unapproved research and can never be reported or published as research data.

° All changes or amendments to the above-referenced protocol require review and approval by the HIC **BEFORE** implementation.

° Adverse Reactions/Unexpected Events (AR/UE) must be submitted on the appropriate form within the timeframe specified in the HIC Policy (http://www.hic.wayne.edu/hicpol.html).

NOTE:

1. Upon notification of an impending regulatory site visit, hold notification, and/or external audit the HIC office must be contacted immediately.
2. Forms should be downloaded from the HIC website at **each** use.

APPENDIX B - A Prospective Study of Punch Biomechanics and Cognitive Function for Amateur Boxers

A prospective study of punch biomechanics and cognitive function for amateur boxers

S Stojsih,[1] M Boitano,[2] M Wilhelm,[1] C Bir[1]

[1] Wayne State University, Detroit, Michigan, USA
[2] McMaster University, Hamilton, Ontario, Canada

Correspondence to:
Dr C Bir, Wayne State University, 818 W Hancock, Detroit, MI 48201-3719, USA; cbir@wayne.edu

Accepted 13 October 2008
Published Online First 19 November 2008

ABSTRACT

Objective: To evaluate several biomechanical factors of the head during a sparring session and their link to cognitive function.

Design: Instrumented Boxing Headgear (IBH) was used for data collection during four 2 min sparring sessions. Neurocognitive assessment was measured using the ImPACT© Concussion management software. A baseline neurocognitive test was obtained from each athlete prior to sparring, two additional tests were obtained and compared with the baseline.

Setting: Male and female amateur boxers.

Participants: Data were collected from 30 male and 30 female amateur boxers.

Main outcome measurements: Head accelerations (translational and rotational), injury severity indexes (Head Injury Criteria (HIC) and Gadd Severity Index (GSI)) and cognitive function scores.

Results: Peak translational and rotational acceleration values were 191 g and 17 156 rad/s^2, respectively, for males and 184 g and 13 113 rad/s^2, respectively, for females. The peak HIC and GSI values for males were 1652 and 2292, respectively, and for females 1079 and 1487, respectively. There was no significant difference in the neurocognitive scores between genders. A decrease was exhibited in the delayed memory postbout scores. All other scores either increased or did not significantly decrease when compared with the baseline.

Conclusions: The majority of impacts experienced by both genders were under the threshold for mild head injury. There was a statistically significant difference between peak translational and rotational acceleration, HIC and GSI when comparing genders. When analysing cognitive functions, there was no statistical difference between genders.

Repetitive head impacts sustained by boxers have become an important discussion in literature due to concern over acute and chronic injuries. A study found that over 70% of acute injuries related to the sport of boxing occur in the head region, with almost half of the injuries to this region being concussions, also referred to as mild traumatic brain injuries (mTBI).[1] Although surrogates have been used to assess the mechanism that causes injuries,[2,4] real-time head acceleration data from the ring and correlation with cognitive function data have yet to be obtained.

Several studies have evaluated the biomechanics of a punch using different surrogate models.[2,4] Atha et al[2] gathered data from a world-ranked British professional heavyweight boxer using a suspended targeted mass with instrumentation. The maximum translational acceleration recorded was 53 g, the peak contact force was 4096 N, and the impact velocity was 8.9 m/s. However, the purpose of the study was to determine the mechanical properties of a boxer's punch, not to observe the effects of a punch in creating an injurious effect. The use of a ballistic pendulum provides force data but does not correlate to head injury risk.

A relationship has been developed between impulse duration and acceleration to assess the risk of head injuries. This relationship is commonly known as the Wayne State Tolerance Curve (WSTC) and is the basis of most head-injury tolerance criteria. The curve indicated a decrease in the tolerable level of acceleration as pulse duration increased. Because the WSTC had various interpretive difficulties, the Gadd Severity Index (GSI) was introduced as a generalisation of the WSTC.[5] A further refinement occurred in 1971 when Versace developed the Head Injury Criterion (HIC), based on the WSTC and GSI.[5,6] Backaitis[7] and Eppinger[8] reported that HIC could be interpreted as a measure of the rate of change in specific kinetic energy imparted to the head, based on the resultant translational acceleration. The well-established HIC threshold of 1000 was developed to identify severe head injuries in automotive safety testing.[9] Recently, an HIC value of 250 was suggested as a threshold for mTBI in professional football.[10]

Although HIC focuses on translational acceleration, forces produced by rapid acceleration or deceleration of the head can cause both translational and rotational movement of the brain, resulting in varying levels of injury. A study by Zhang et al[11] proposed thresholds for translational and rotational acceleration based on a finite element model of the brain. The threshold established that a translational and rotational acceleration of 66 g and 4600 rad/s^2 (25% probability), 82 g and 5900 rad/s^2 (50% probability), and 106 g and 7900 rad/s^2 (80% probability), respectively, would result in brain injury.

In a study correlating these injury parameters to impacts from Olympic boxers, Walilko et al[4] evaluated the biomechanics of a punch to the jaw to determine the risk of head injury from translational and rotational accelerations using a Hybrid III anthropomorphic head. The translational acceleration was reported to be 58 (SD 13) g, the rotational acceleration was 6343 (1789) rad/s^2, and the HIC was 71 (49). Although providing some preliminary data, this study is limited due to the lack of biofidelity of the jaw and Hybrid III headform for such an application.

Given advances in wireless technology, the collection of real-time data without game time

Original article

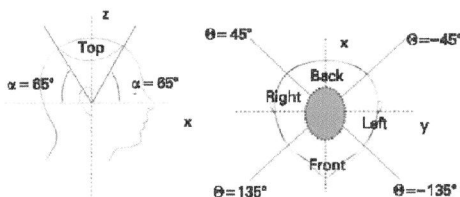

Figure 1 General impact locations.

interference is now possible. Simbex (Lebanon, New Hampshire) developed the Head Impact Telemetry (HIT) system to collect real-time head acceleration data during sporting activities. The system has been validated and utilised in various sports, specifically football.[12,13] The use of such technology within the sport of boxing will allow for more precise analyses of both the impact and resulting outcome. The goal of the current study was to collect real-time head acceleration data from amateur boxers and document any resulting cognitive changes.

METHODS
Sample population
A total of 30 male and 30 female amateur boxers consented to participate. The mean age of the male athletes was 22 years with a mean experience level of 6 years, and the mean age of the female athletes was 24 years with a mean experience of 3 years at the amateur level. Approval was garnered from the Wayne State University Human Investigation Committee prior to testing, with all subjects consenting to participate prior to testing.

Impact boxing headgear data collection
The Impact Boxing Headgear (IBH), a modification of the HIT system, is a wireless system that provides real-time data to a ringside receiver and laptop computer. The system was developed by Simbex and validated prior to testing.[14] Each headgear consists of 12 single axis linear accelerometers, a wireless transceiver, onboard memory and data-acquisition capabilities (1000 Hz). For each impact the IBH data were collected over a 40 ms time window (8 ms pretrigger and 32 ms post-trigger) when any accelerometer exceeded $9.6\,g$. The acceleration data are time stamped and wirelessly transmitted to the receiver interfaced with a laptop computer. If wireless communication is not present, the onboard memory within the headgear stores up to 100 impacts, and data are downloaded once communication has been restored.

Boxers were instructed to spar for four 2 min rounds with an opponent of the same weight class and gender. Impact data from the headgear were postprocessed by researchers at Simbex using an algorithm to calculate translational head acceleration, rotational head acceleration and impact location.[14] Impact locations (front, back, top, right and left) were determined using the azimuth (θ) and elevation (α) recorded for each impact (fig 1).[15] Two impact severity scores that relate head acceleration to risk of injury, HIC and GSI, were also calculated.[5,6]

Neurocognitive assessment data collection
Within 24 h prior to the sparring session, each boxer completed baseline testing using the ImPACT© Version 5.0 cognitive software.[16] Postbout tests were obtained within 30 min and 24 h following the sparring session. Each athlete performed the brief computerised test on a laptop computer with a mouse in a quiet area of the boxing facility.

The scores that resulted from the modules during the postbout tests were compared with the module results from the baseline test. From this comparison, several scores were generated to assess the boxer's memory, attention, problem solving and reaction time.

STATISTICAL ANALYSIS
The IBH and cognitive function data were analysed using Statistical Package for Social Sciences (SPSS) version 16.0.2. A MANOVA was conducted when comparing the IBH data; however, violations of the normality assumption occurred, and non-parametric tests (Mann–Whitney) were used to make the comparison. The comparison of the number of impacts sustained between genders was analysed using a t test. A one-way ANOVA was used for the IBH impact location data to determine the equality of the means without grouping by gender. For the cognitive function data, a repeated-measures ANOVA was applied to analyse scores between and within gender groups. If a violation of the normality occurred, the non-parametric Mann–Whitney test for between-group comparisons and Wilcoxon signed ranks test for within-group comparisons were utilised. For all tests with multiple comparisons, Bonferroni adjustments were made to decrease the number of Type I errors. Pearson correlations were conducted on the peak values for the translational and rotational acceleration, HIC, GSI and number of impacts versus ImPACT subscores to determine if there were any significant relationships.

RESULTS
Impact boxing headgear
Five participants withdrew from the study prior to the sparring session because cheek protectors were not an option on the instrumented headgear; therefore, the IBH data (tables 1, 2) included 55 participants with 1930 impacts. Twenty-seven of the participants were males with 1128 impacts (42 impacts/boxer), and the remaining 28 participants were females with 802 impacts (29 impacts/boxer).

No significant difference was found for the mean acceleration and injury severity scores when comparing gender groups using the non-parametric Mann–Whitney test. The peak HIC, GSI, translational acceleration and rotational acceleration values were also compared by gender groups. Male boxers experienced a significantly higher peak translational acceleration ($p = 0.006$),

Table 1 Descriptive statistics for mean Instrumented Boxing Headgear impact data

	No of impacts*	Head Injury Criteria 15	Gadd Severity Index	Translational peak (g)	Rotational peak (rad/s²)
Male	42 (27)	43 (100)	66 (148)	30 (21)	2571 (1892)
Female	29 (18)	32 (66)	49 (93)	28 (17)	2533 (1524)

*p<0.05.

Table 2 Descriptive statistics for peak Instrumented Boxing Headgear impact data

	No of impacts	Head Injury Criteria 15*	Gadd Severity Index*	Translational peak (g)*	Rotational peak (rad/s²)*
Male	104	1652	2292	191	17 156
Female	83	1079	1487	184	13 113

*$p<0.05$.

HIC ($p=0.005$) and GSI ($p=0.005$) when compared with female boxers with an adjusted alpha level of $\alpha = 0.0125$. The peak rotational accelerations exhibited a mild level of significance ($p=0.013$). Additionally, a t test was performed to compare the mean number of impacts between gender groups. The male boxers had a significantly higher number of impacts (41.8 impacts/boxer) when compared with the female boxers (28.6 impacts/boxer) ($p=0.04$) (table 1).

Figures 2-4 illustrate that the majority of the impacts sustained by the boxers were below the 25% probability threshold for brain injury established by Zhang et al.[11] Combining the male and female data, 94.8% of the impacts were under the translational acceleration threshold, and 89.6% of the impacts were under the rotational acceleration threshold. The percentage of impacts experienced by both genders that were under the mTBI threshold of 250, suggested by Pellman et al,[10] was 97.8%.

Figure 5 illustrates the total number of impacts that were sustained by all of the boxers grouped by location. A one-way ANOVA was used to compare the total number of impacts recorded for each region of the head. With an adjusted alpha value, $\alpha = 0.0125$, the total number of impacts to the front region of the head (56%) (n=1930) was significantly higher when compared with the other locations ($p=0.000$): left (17%), right (14%), back (11%) and top (2%). Although the male boxers experienced a higher number of impacts, the impact location trend was comparable for both genders.

The mean accelerations and HIC scores were compared by general impact location using the non-parametric Mann-Whitney test. No significant difference was observed between gender groups. Impacts to the front and top locations of the head were statistically significant when compared with the other locations (table 3). The mean translational acceleration for the front was significantly lower compared with the back ($p=0.000$), right ($p=0.009$) and left ($p=0.008$) regions, the mean rotational acceleration was significantly lower compared with the three regions ($p=0.000$) as well, and the mean HIC score was significantly lower compared with the back ($p=0.011$) and left ($p=0.007$) regions. The mean translational acceleration and mean HIC score for the top location were significantly lower when compared with the back, right and left regions ($p=0.000$). Additionally, the mean rotational acceleration was significantly lower than the back ($p=0.012$) and left ($p=0.013$) regions in comparison with the top location. The values remain significant with an adjusted alpha value of $\alpha = 0.0167$ due to repeated comparisons.

Figure 6 depicts a graph of the rotational and translational accelerations for each impact. The impacts are labelled by the general location. The impacts with the highest rotational and translational accelerations were front impacts. The shaded box in the lower left corner of the graph illustrates the impacts that are below the 25% probability of brain damage established by Zhang et al.[11]

Neurocognitive assessment

Five athletes were unable to complete the testing series for various reasons (inability to locate the athletes following the session and cooperation issues); therefore, complete cognitive data sets were collected from 55 boxers, 26 males and 29 females (table 4).

Both parametric and non-parametric tests were utilised when appropriate and exhibited no significant difference when comparing gender groups. However, a significant decrease was reported for the delayed memory postscores when analysing the data using repeated-measures ANOVA. A pairwise comparison of the three time points for delayed memory revealed significance between the baseline test and post-test for both males and females ($p=0.000$) with an adjusted alpha value for multiple tests, $\alpha = 0.025$. The other scores either increased following the sparring session or did not significantly decrease when compared with the baseline tests. In addition, Pearson correlations between the head accelerations, HIC, number of impacts and cognitive scores were also investigated, but the results were not clinically significant.

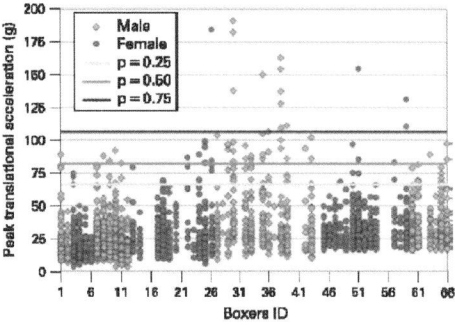

Figure 2 Male and female peak translational acceleration (g).

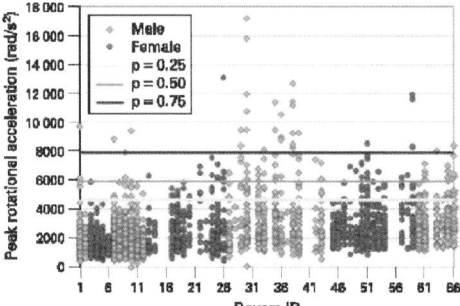

Figure 3 Male and female peak rotational acceleration (rad/s²).

Original article

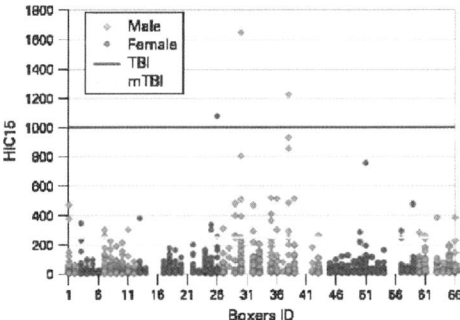

Figure 4 Male and female Head Injury Criteria scores. mTBI, Mild head injury or concussion; TBI, Severe head injury.

Table 3 General locations and corresponding mean accelerations and injury severity

	Translational acceleration (g)	Rotational acceleration (rad/s²)	Head Injury Criteria
Front	27 (18)*	2307 (1597)*	33 (81)†
Right	31 (19)	2809 (1705)	43 (78)
Left	32 (22)	2898 (1874)	47 (97)
Top	20 (14)*	2251 (1410)†	16 (27)*
Back	34 (25)	3004 (1982)	52 (116)

*$p<0.05$.
†Mean scores were not significant when comparing the front and top to the right values but were significant when compared with the back and left values.

DISCUSSION

The purpose of this study was to measure and analyse several biomechanical factors (translational acceleration, rotational acceleration, HIC, GSI and impact location) during sparring sessions and cognitive functioning of the athletes following the activity. Amateur boxers volunteered for the study from various gyms, clubs and training camps. The IBH system was utilised to collect real-time head impact data in the ring, while neurocognitive functions were assessed prior to sparring and at two time points following sparring sessions.

The current research revealed the mean magnitude of the impacts, obtained by the IBH system, to be lower than previously reported in the literature (table 5). Data from previously published literature were obtained when boxers impacted a surrogate at maximum impact speeds. The current study collected data during sparring sessions, and so the biomechanical factors observed may be lower than what would be recorded during competitive bouts. Further research should be conducted to determine whether competition would significantly increase the impacts experienced, and ultimately the cognitive function of the athletes. Although the sparring scenario provides the ability to have a more controlled study, competitive bouts would provide more realistic data. The majority of the impacts sustained in this study were subconcussive, and no concussions were noted in any of the participants following the sparring sessions. It is anticipated that more concussive events would be captured in a competition setting.

Additionally, the general location of each impact was determined by the IBH system. Research has indicated that acceleration, duration and direction of the impact load may influence the outcome of an impact to the head.[6 10 11 17 20] More frequently, impacts in the lateral direction have been documented to result in brain injury.[17 20] The current study revealed that impacts to either the side or back of the head exhibited, on average, significantly higher accelerations and HIC scores ($p<0.05$) (table 3). The impacts to the front region of the head produced significantly lower mean acceleration values which may be a result of specific training activities. Some athletes focus on building their cervical neck muscles to aid in the incidence or severity of concussion injury by potentially decreasing head acceleration.[21] An additional explanation for the low head accelerations could be the frequency of the impacts to the front region of the head. Over half of all the impacts sustained were to the front region, indicating that athletes may be more prepared for those impacts resulting in reduced head accelerations.

While there are some data investigating the punch forces of male boxers,[2 4] the literature regarding female boxers is limited. This study provides one of the first analyses of real-time punch force data and cognitive function in female amateur boxers along with a comparison of the male and female data. When

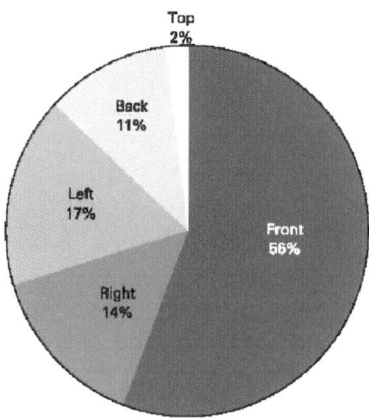

Figure 5 General locations for each impact sustained.

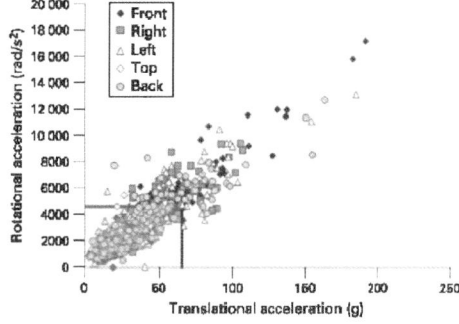

Figure 6 Rotational and translational accelerations of each impact based on general location.

Table 4 Mean ImPACT scores for baseline, post and 24 h postbout tests

	Baseline		Post		24 h post	
	Male	Female	Male	Female	Male	Female
Verbal memory	80 (10)	80 (10)	81 (10)	82 (11)	82 (11)	84 (9)
Visual memory	68 (13)	65 (13)	70 (13)	61 (14)	69 (14)	69 (13)
Visual motor speed	33.7 (8.8)	32.8 (8.1)	34.9 (8.4)	37.4 (7.6)	35.3 (9.3)	37.0 (7.9)
Reaction time	0.61 (0.09)	0.64 (0.16)	0.57 (0.11)	0.60 (0.12)	0.60 (0.08)	0.59 (0.10)
Immediate memory	0.87 (0.05)	0.85 (0.07)	0.84 (0.09)	0.83 (0.08)	0.86 (0.09)	0.86 (0.06)
Delayed memory	0.80 (0.06)	0.79 (0.07)	0.73 (0.14)*	0.74 (0.09)*	0.75 (0.14)	0.76 (0.08)
Working memory	0.66 (0.15)	0.64 (0.14)	0.72 (0.11)	0.67 (0.14)	0.72 (0.14)	0.73 (0.15)

*$p<0.05$ comparison of post-tests with baseline test.

analysing the IBH impact data, the male boxers had significantly higher ($p<0.05$) peak values when compared with the females. In addition, the frequency of impacts sustained by the male boxers was significantly higher ($p<0.05$) when compared with the female boxers. However, a significant difference was not established when comparing mean translational and rotational accelerations, HIC and GSI between genders (table 1). On average, the male boxers experienced more impacts, but the magnitude of the impacts for both genders was similar. Comparison of the cognitive function data between genders proved that there was no significant difference in memory, attention, reaction time and problem solving following the sparring sessions.

Head accelerations and injury severity scores obtained from each impact during the sparring proved that the majority of the impacts were below suggested injury thresholds.[11] The neurocognitive tests indicated that the athletes had difficulties retaining information during the postsparring test as indicated in a significant decrease in the delayed memory scores. This finding indicates that immediately after a boxer spars, retention of new information is compromised. Twenty four hours following the bout, the delayed memory score was still lower than the baseline; however, it was not significant. The present results compliment the results yielded in a study by Heilbronner et al[22] where neuropsychological tests were administered to 26 amateur boxers. Comparison of test scores before and after a single sparring session showed a deficit in verbal memory and incidental memory in the amateur boxers.

In contrast, other studies have found no relationship between amateur boxing and cognitive dysfunction. Moriarty et al[23] followed 82 amateur boxers in a 7-day tournament and found no evidence of cognitive dysfunction in the immediate postbout period. In a 9-year prospective study of amateur boxers, Porter[24] found that the boxers exhibited no evidence of neuropsychological deterioration. Other studies also support this conclusion.[25 26] Although Butler[16] found no sign of neuropsychological dysfunction, it was suggested that a long amateur career might reduce fine motor movements. More extensive data are needed over a longer time line to determine the potential effects of repetitive concussive and subconcussive head impacts in amateur boxers.

This study represents the first in-ring collection of impact data for both males and females. These findings are an important contribution to both impact biomechanics and cognitive impairment research. Further efforts will enhance the body of knowledge related to the biomechanics of boxing and sports-related brain injury. It is critical to determine thresholds of injury so that protective measures, including headgear and gloves, may be properly evaluated.

Acknowledgements: The National Operating Committee on Standards for Athletic Equipment provided funding for this research project. Impact Boxing Headgear was developed for this study by Simbex, and the IBH data were postprocessed by J Beckwith of Simbex. K Podell assisted in the postprocessing of the neurocognitive data. Boxers from USA boxing, U of M, the Armed Forces, Ramos Boxing Gym, Zarzamora Street Gym, Windsor Boxing Club and Border City Boxing Gym volunteered their time to participate in the study. E Hanlon, C Schreiner, R Bolander and O Pinto Neto assisted in data collection for the study. Statistical analysis was completed by B Ozkan, from Wayne State University.

Funding: The National Operating Committee on Standards for Athletic Equipment provided funding for this research project.

Competing interests: None.

Ethics approval: Ethics approval was provided by Wayne State University Human Investigation Committee.

REFERENCES

1. Zazryn TR, Cameron P, McCrory P. A prospective cohort study of injury in amateur and professional boxing. Br J Sports Med 2006;40:670–4.
2. Atha J, Yeadon MR, Sandover J, et al. The damaging punch. BMJ 1985;291:1756–7.
3. Smith MS, Dyson RJ, Hale T, et al. Development of a boxing dynamometer and its punch force discrimination efficacy. J Sports Sci 2000;18:445–50.
4. Walilko TJ, Viano DC, Bir CA. Biomechanics of the head for Olympic boxer punches to the face. Br J Sports Med 2005;39:710–19.
5. McElhaney JH, Roberts V, Hilyard J. Handbook of human tolerance. Tsukuba, Japan: Automobile Research Institute, 1976:788–91.
6. Versace J. A review of the severity index. In: Proceedings of the 15th Stapp Car Crash Conference, 1971. SAE paper 710881:771–96.
7. Backaitis S. The head injury criterion. Head and neck injury criteria: a consensus workshop. Washington: US Department of Transportation, 1981:175–7.
8. Eppinger R. Discussion of injury criteria. Head and neck injury criteria: a consensus workshop. Washington: US Department of Transportation, 1981:204–49.
9. Holbourn A. Mechanics of head injury. Lancet 1943;2:438–41.
10. Pellman EJ, Viano DC, Tucker AM, et al. Concussion in professional football. Reconstruction of game impacts and injuries. Neurosurgery 2003;53:799–812.
11. Zhang L, Yang KH, King AI. A proposed injury threshold for mild traumatic brain injury. J Biomech Eng 2004;126:226–36.
12. Brolinson P, Manoogian S, McNeely D, et al. Analysis of linear head accelerations from collegiate football impacts. Curr Sports Med Rep 2006;5:23–8.
13. Duma S, Manoogian SJ, Bussone WR, et al. Analysis of real-time head accelerations in collegiate football players. Clin J Sport Med 2005;15:3–8.
14. Beckwith JG, Chu JJ, Greenwald RM. Validation of a noninvasive system for measuring head acceleration for use during boxing competition. J Appl Biomech 2007;23:238–44.
15. Crisco J, Chu J, Greenwald R. An algorithm for estimating acceleration magnitude and impact location using multiple nonorthogonal single-axis accelerometers. J Biomech Eng 2004;126:849–54.
16. ImPACT Applications Inc. Website. http://www.impacttest.com (accessed 18 July 2008).
17. Delaney J, Puni V, Rouah F. Mechanisms of injury for concussions in university football, ice hockey, and soccer. A pilot study. Clin J Sport Med 2006;16:162–5.
18. Kleiven S. Influence of impact direction on the human head in prediction of subdural hematoma. J Neurotrauma 2003;20:365–79.

Table 5 Comparison of data found in literature for male boxers

	Translational acceleration (g)	Rotational acceleration (rad/s^2)	Head Injury Criteria
Current study	30 (21)	2571 (1852)	43 (100)
Atha et al[2]	53	–	–
Walilko et al[4]	58 (13)	6343 (1789)	71 (49)

Original article

19. **Ommaya A**, Gennarelli T. Cerebral concussion and traumatic unconsciousness. Correlation of experimental and clinical observations of blunt head injuries. *Brain* 1974;**97**:633–54.
20. **Zhang L**, Yang K, King A. Comparison of brain responses between frontal and lateral impacts by finite element modeling. *J Neurotrauma* 2001;**18**:21–30.
21. **Cross K**, Serenelli C. Training and equipment to prevent athletic head and neck injuries. *Clin Sports Med* 2003;**22**:639–62.
22. **Heilbronner R**, Henry G, Carson-Brewer M. Neuropsychologic test performance in amateur boxers. *Am J Sports Med* 1991;**19**:376–80.
23. **Moriarity J**, Collie A, Olson D, et al. A prospective controlled study of cognitive function during an amateur boxing tournament. *Neurology* 2004;**62**:1497–502.
24. **Porter M**. A 9-year controlled prospective neuropsychologic assessment of amateur boxing. *Clin J Sport Med* 2003;**13**:339–52.
25. **Brooks N**, Kupshik G, Wilson L, et al. A neuropsychological study of active amateur boxers. *J Neurol Neurosurg Psychiatry* 1987;**50**:997–1000.
26. **Butler R**. Neuropsychological investigation of amateur boxers. *Br J Sports Med* 1994;**28**:187–90.

APPENDIX C – Standardized Assessment of Concussion (SAC) Forms A and B

STANDARDIZED ASSESSMENT OF CONCUSSION (SAC)
Form A

NAME: _____
TEAM: _____ EXAMINER: _____
DATE OF EXAM: _____ TIME: _____
EXAM (Circle One): BLINE INJURY FOLLOW-UP: _____

ORIENTATION 1 point for each correct answer
What Month is it?	0 1	Today's Date?	0 1
Day of the Week?	0 1	The Year?	0 1
Current Time (within 1 hr)	0 1		

ORIENTATION TOTAL SCORE /5

IMMEDIATE MEMORY
Complete all 3 trials regardless of score on trial 1 & 2. 1 pt for each correct response. Total score equals sum across all 3 trials.

LIST	TRIAL 1	TRIAL 2	TRIAL 3
ELBOW	0 1	0 1	0 1
APPLE	0 1	0 1	0 1
CARPET	0 1	0 1	0 1
SADDLE	0 1	0 1	0 1
BUBBLE	0 1	0 1	0 1
TOTAL			

IMMEDIATE MEMORY TOTAL SCORE /15

Do not inform the subject that delayed recall will be tested.

EXERTIONAL MANEUVERS (when appropriate)
5 Jumping Jacks, 5 Push-Ups, 5 Sit-ups, 5 Knee Bends

NEUROLOGIC SCREENING

LOSS OF CONSCIOUSNESS/ WITNESSED UNRESPONSIVENESS	☐ No Length:	☐ Yes
POST-TRAUMATIC AMNESIA? Poor recall of events after injury	☐ No Length	☐ Yes
RETROGRADE AMNESIA? Poor recall of events before injury	☐ No Length	☐ Yes
	NORMAL	ABNORMAL
STRENGTH Right Upper Extremity Left Upper Extremity Right Lower Extremity Left Lower Extremity	☐ ☐ ☐ ☐	☐ ☐ ☐ ☐
SENSATION - examples: FINGER-TO-NOSE/ROMBERG	☐	☐
COORDINATION - examples: TANDEM GAIT/FINGER-NOSE-FINGER	☐	☐

Please see reverse side for important user information

CONCENTRATION
Digits Backward: If correct, go to next string length. If incorrect, read trial 2. 1 pt possible for each string length. Stop after incorrect on both trials.

4-9-3	6-2-9	0 1
3-8-1-4	3-2-7-9	0 1
6-2-9-7-1	1-5-2-8-6	0 1
7-1-8-4-6-2	5-3-9-1-4-8	0 1

Months in Reverse Order 1 pt for entire sequence correct
Dec-Nov-Oct-Sep-Aug-Jul-Jun-May-Apr-Mar-Feb-Jan   0 1

CONCENTRATION TOTAL SCORE /5

DELAYED RECALL Circle and award 1 point for each word correctly recalled

ELBOW   APPLE   CARPET   SADDLE   BUBBLE

DELAYED RECALL TOTAL SCORE /5

SAC SCORING SUMMARY

ORIENTATION	/5
IMMEDIATE MEMORY	/15
CONCENTRATION	/5
DELAYED RECALL	/5
SAC TOTAL SCORE	/30

**Exertional Maneuvers & Neurologic Screening are important for examination, but not incorporated into SAC Total Score.

IMPORTANT USER INFORMATION: The SAC is a complement to, not a substitute for, a clinical examination by a physician, athletic trainer or other qualified health provider. The SAC is not intended as a stand-alone method of concussion assessment or return-to-play decision-making. SAC results should be complemented by all aspects of injury evaluation, and all clinical information should be considered in the assessment and management of concussion. The SAC is not intended as a substitute for formal neurologic or neuropsychological evaluation of an injured person. The SAC record form (or exam card) is not to be used without a thorough understanding of the contents of the SAC manual for administration, scoring and interpretation. The standardization, reliability and validity of the SAC may be significantly compromised by any user who is not familiar with the contents of the SAC manual. All SAC materials are protected by copyright and should not be circulated via photocopy or any other medium without written consent from the authors. Please review the 'Important Warning and Disclaimer' at the front of the SAC manual for additional important information incorporated herein by reference.

Copyright ©2000 by McCrea, Kelly and Randolph. All rights reserved. May not be reproduced in whole or in part in any form or by any means without written permission from the authors. This form is printed in blue ink on white paper. Any other version is unauthorized. Doc. 503239 RevA

STANDARDIZED ASSESSMENT OF CONCUSSION (SAC)
Form B

NAME: _____
TEAM: _____ EXAMINER: _____
DATE OF EXAM: _____ TIME: _____
EXAM (Circle One): BLINE INJURY FOLLOW-UP:

ORIENTATION 1 point for each correct answer.

What Month is it?	0 1	Today's Date?	0 1	
Day of the Week?	0 1	The Year?	0 1	
Current Time (within 1 hr)	0 1			

ORIENTATION TOTAL SCORE	/5

IMMEDIATE MEMORY
Complete all 3 trials regardless of score on trial 1 & 2. 1 pt. for each correct response. Total score equals sum across all 3 trials.

LIST	TRIAL 1	TRIAL 2	TRIAL 3
CANDLE	0 1	0 1	0 1
PAPER	0 1	0 1	0 1
SUGAR	0 1	0 1	0 1
SANDWICH	0 1	0 1	0 1
WAGON	0 1	0 1	0 1
TOTAL			

IMMEDIATE MEMORY TOTAL SCORE	/15

Do not inform the subject that delayed recall will be tested.

EXERTIONAL MANEUVERS (when appropriate)
5 Jumping Jacks, 5 Push-Ups, 5 Sit-ups, 5 Knee Bends

NEUROLOGIC SCREENING

LOSS OF CONSCIOUSNESS/ WITNESSED UNRESPONSIVENESS	☐ No Length:	☐ Yes
POST-TRAUMATIC AMNESIA? Poor recall of events after injury	☐ No Length:	☐ Yes
RETROGRADE AMNESIA? Poor recall of events before injury	☐ No Length:	☐ Yes

	NORMAL	ABNORMAL
STRENGTH Right Upper Extremity Left Upper Extremity Right Lower Extremity Left Lower Extremity	☐ ☐ ☐ ☐	☐ ☐ ☐ ☐
SENSATION - examples: FINGER-TO-NOSE/ROMBERG	☐	☐
COORDINATION - examples: TANDEM GAIT/FINGER-NOSE-FINGER	☐	☐

Please see reverse side for important user information

CONCENTRATION
Digits Backward: If correct, go to next string length. If incorrect, read trial 2. 1 pt. possible for each string length. Stop after incorrect on both trials.

5-2-8	4-1-5	0 1
1-7-9-5	4-9-6-8	0 1
4-8-5-2-7	6-1-8-4-3	0 1
8-3-1-9-6-4	7-2-4-8-5-6	0 1

Months in Reverse Order 1 pt. for entire sequence correct
Dec-Nov-Oct-Sept-Aug-Jul-Jun-May-Apr-Mar-Feb-Jan   0 1

CONCENTRATION TOTAL SCORE	/5

DELAYED RECALL Circle and award 1 point for each word correctly recalled

CANDLE   PAPER   SUGAR   SANDWICH   WAGON

DELAYED RECALL TOTAL SCORE	/5

SAC SCORING SUMMARY

ORIENTATION	/ 5
IMMEDIATE MEMORY	/ 15
CONCENTRATION	/ 5
DELAYED RECALL	/ 5
SAC TOTAL SCORE	/ 30

**Exertional Maneuvers & Neurologic Screening are important for examination, but not incorporated into SAC Total Score

IMPORTANT USER INFORMATION: The SAC is a complement to, not a substitute for, a clinical examination by a physician, athletic trainer or other qualified health provider. The SAC is not intended as a stand-alone method of concussion assessment or return-to-play decision-making. SAC results should be complemented by all aspects of injury evaluation, and all clinical information should be considered in the assessment and management of concussion. The SAC is not intended as a substitute for formal neurologic or neuropsychological evaluation of an injured person. The SAC record form (or exam card) is not to be used without a thorough understanding of the contents of the SAC manual for administration, scoring and interpretation. The standardization, reliability and validity of the SAC may be significantly compromised by any user who is not familiar with the contents of the SAC manual. All SAC materials are protected by copyright and should not be circulated via photocopy or any other medium without written consent from the authors. Please review the "Important Warning and Disclaimer" at the front of the SAC manual for additional important information incorporated herein by reference.

Copyright ©2000 by McCrea, Kelly and Randolph. All rights reserved. May not be reproduced in whole or in part in any form or by any means without written permission from the authors. This form is printed in red ink on white paper. Any other version is unauthorized. Doc 503240 RevA

REFERENCES

AAN Quality Standards Committee, 1997. Practice parameter: the management of concussion in sports (summary statement). Report of the Quality Standards Subcommittee Neurology 48, 581-587.

Atha J., Yeadon M.R., et al., 1985. The damaging punch. British Medical Journal 291, 1756-1757.

Auer L., 1989. Epidural and subdural hematoma. Handbook of clinical neurology. P. Vinken, G. Bruyn and H. Klawans. Amsterdam, Elsevier Science B.V.

Backaitis S., 1981. The head injury criterion. Head and neck criteria: a consensus workshop. US Department of Transportation 175-177.

Bailes J. and Cantu R., 2001. Head injury in athletes. Neurosurgery 48(1), 26-45.

Barnes B.C., Cooper L., et al., 1998. Concussion history in elite male and female soccer players. The American Journal of Sports Medicine 26(3), 433-438.

Beckwith J., Chu J., et al., 2007. Validation of a Noninvasive System for Measuring Head Acceleration for Use During Boxing Competition. Journal of Applied Biomechanics 23, 238-244.

Bianco M., Pannozzo A., et al., 2005. Medical survey of female boxing in Italy 2002-2003. Br. J. Sports Med. 39, 532-536.

Boden B.P., Kirkendall D.T., et al., 1998. Concussion incidence in elite college soccer players. The American Journal of Sports Medicine 26(2), 238-241.

Brolinson P., Manoogian S., et al., 2006. Analysis of Linear Head Accelerations from Collegiate Football Impacts. Current Sports Medicine Reports 5, 23-28.

Brooks N., Kupshik G., et al., 1987. A neuropsychological study of active amateur boxers Journal of neurology, neurosurgery, and psychiatry 50, 997-1000.

Butler R., 1994. Neuropsychological investigation of amateur boxers. Br. J. Sports Med. 28, 187-190.

Cantu R., 1996. Head injuries in sport. Br J Sports Med 30, 289-296.

Cantu R., 1998. Second-Impact Syndrome Clinics in Sports Medicine 17(1), 37-44.

Cantu R. and Mueller F., 2003. Brain injury-related fatalities in American football, 1945-1999. Neurosurgery 52(4), 852-3.

Chu J., Beckwith J., et al., 2006. A novel algorithm to measure linear and rotational head acceleration using single-axis accelerometers In Proceedings of Conference proceedings of the 5th World Congress of Biomechanics. Munich, Germany.

Collins M., Grindel S., et al., 1999. Relationship between concussion and neuropsychological performance in college football players. JAMA 282(10), 964-970.

Corsellis J., 1989. Boxing and the brain. Br Med J 298, 105-9.

Corsellis J., Bruton C., et al., 1973. The aftermath of boxing. Psychol Med 3, 270-303.

Covassin T., Swanik C.B., et al., 2003. Sex difference and the incidence of concussions among collegiate athletes. Journal of athletic training 38(3), 238-244.

Crisco J., Chu J., et al., 2004. An algorithm for estimating acceleration magnitude and impact location using multiple nonorthogonal single-axis accelerometers Journal of Biomechanical Engineering 126, 849-854.

Cross K. and Serenelli C., 2003. Training and equipment to prevent athletic head and neck injuries. Clin Sports Med 22, 639-667.

Dau N., Chein H., et al., 2006. Effectiveness of Boxing Headgear for Limiting Injury. American Society of Biomechanics.

De Kruijk J., Twijnstra A., et al., 2001. Diagnostic criteria and differential diagnosis of mild traumatic brain injury. Brain Injury 15(2), 99-106.

Delaney J., Puni V., et al., 2006. Mechanisms of injury for concussions in university football, ice hockey, and soccer: A pilot study. Clin J Sport Med 16, 162-165.

Duma S., Manoogian S., et al., 2005. Analysis of real-time head accelerations in collegiate football players. Clin J Sport Med 15, 3-8.

Eppinger R., 1981. Discussion of injury criteria. Head and neck injury criteria: a consensus workshop. US Department of Transportation, 204-249.

Field M., Collins M., et al., 2003. Does age play a role in recovery from sport-related concussion? A comparison of high school and collegiate athletes. The Journal of Pediatrics, 546-553.

Funk J., Duma S., et al., 2007. Biomechanical risk estimates for mild traumatic brain injury. In Proceedings of 51st Annual Proceedings of the Association for the Advancement of Automotive Medicine. Melbourne, Australia

Gadd C., 1966. Use of a Weighted-Impulse Criterion for Estimating Injury Hazard. In Proceedings of 10th Stapp Car Crash Conference. SAE Paper No. 660793.

Gaetz M., Goodman D., et al., 2000. Electrophysiological evidence for the cumulative effects of concussion. Brain Injury 14, 1077-1088.

Garfield J., 2002. Acute subdural haematoma in a boxer. British Journal of Neurosurgery 16(2), 96-101.

Gennarelli T., Ommaya A., et al., 1971. Comaprison of rotaional and translational head motions in experimental cerebral concussion. Proc 15th Stapp Car Crash Conference SAE P-39, 797-803.

Gennarelli T., Thibault L., et al., 1972. Pathophysiological responses to rotational and translational accelerations of the head. Proc 16th Stapp Car Crash Conference SAE Paper No. 720970.

Gerberding J. and Binder S., 2003. Report to Congress on mild traumatic brain injury in the United States: Steps to prevent a serious public health problem, National Center for Injury Prevention and Control.

Granacher Jr. R., 2008. Traumatic brain injury: Methods for clinical and forensic neuropsychiatric assessment Boca Raton, Taylor & Francis Group.

Gronwall D. and Wrightson P., 1975. Cumulative effect of concussion. The Lancet, 995-997.

Gurdjian E. and Lissner H., 1961. Photoelastic confirmation of the presence of shear strains at the conjunction in closed head injury J Neurosurg 18, 58-60.

Gurdjian E., Webster J., *et al.*, 1955. Observations on the mechanism of brain concussion, contusion, and laceration. Surg Gynec Obstet 101, 680-690.

Gurdjian E.W., JE, 1945. Linear acceleration causing shear in the brain stem in trauma of the central nervous system. Mental Adv Dis 24, 28.

Guskiewicz K., McCrea M., *et al.*, 2003. Cumulative effects associated with recurrent concussion in collegiate football players: The NCAA concussion study. JAMA 290(19), 2549-2555.

Haglund Y. and Eriksson E., 1993. Does amateur boxing lead to chronic brain damage? The American Journal of Sports Medicine 21(1), 97-109.

Hammeke T. and Gennarelli T., 2003. Traumatic brain injury. Neuropsychiatry. R. Schiffer, S. Rao and B. Fogel. Philadelphia, Lippincott Williams & Wilkins: 1168-1190.

Heilbronner R., Bush S., *et al.*, 2009. Neuropsychological consequences of boxing and recommendations to improve safety: A National Academy of Neuropsychology education paper. Archives of Clinical Neuropsychology 24, 11-19.

Heilbronner R., Henry G., *et al.*, 1991. Neuropsychologic test performance in amateur boxers Am J Sports Med 19(4), 376-380.

Hillary F., Mann C., *et al.*, 2002. Increased risk for concussion in female athletes. In Proceedings of 2002 NAN Conference

Holbourn A., 1943. Mechanics of head injury, Lancet.

Ingebrigtsen T. and Rommer B., 2002. Biochemical serum markers of traumatic brain injury. Journal of Trauma 52(4), 798-808.

Iverson G., Brooks B., et al., 2006. No cumulative effects for one or two previous concussions British J of Sport Med 40, 72-75.

Iverson G., Gaetz M., et al., 2003. Cumulative effects of concussion in amateur athletes. Brain Injury 18(5), 433-443.

Jordan B., Relkin N., et al., 1997. Apolipoprotein E4 associated with chronic traumatic brain injury in boxing. JAMA 278(2), 136-40.

Jordan B., Voy R., et al., 1990. Amateur boxing injuries at the United States Olympic Training Center The Physician and Sports Medicine 18, 81-90.

King A., Yang K., et al., 2003. Is head injury caused by linear or angular acceleration? IRCOBI Conference. Lisbon.

Kleiven S., 2003. Influence of impact direction on the human head in prediction of subdural hematoma. Journal of Neurotrauma 20(4), 365-379.

Kutner K., Erlanger D., et al., 2000. Lower cognitive performance of older football players possessing Apolipoprotein E epsilon 4 Neurosurgery 47(3), 651-658.

Lipsky R., Sparling M., et al., 2005. Association of COMT Val158Met genotype with executive functioning following traumatic brain injury J Neurpsychiatry Clin Neurosci 17(4), 465-471.

Loosemore M., Knowles C., et al., 2007. Amateur boxing and risk of chronic traumatic brain injury: systematic review of observational studies. BMJ.

Lovell M., Collins M., et al., 2004. Grade 1 or 'Ding' concussions in high school athletes. American Journal of Sports Medicine 32.

Lovell M. and West R., 2005. Gender differences regarding concussions in high school and collegiate athletes In Proceedings of 2005 American Academy of Orthopedic Surgeons Annual Meeting. Washington, DC.

Lowenhielm P., 1975. Mathematical simulation of gliding contusions J Biomechanics 8, 351-356.

Macciocchi S., Barth J., et al., 2001. Multiple concussions and neuropsychological functioning in collegiate football players. Journal of athletic training 36(3), 303-306.

Martland H., 1928. Punch drunk. JAMA 91, 1103-1107.

Matser E., Kessels A., et al., 2000. Acute traumatic brain injury in amateur boxing The Physician and Sports Medicine 28, 87-92.

Matser J., Kessels A., et al., 1998. Chronic traumatic brain injury in professional soccer players. Neurology 51(3), 791-6.

McCrea M., 2001. Standardized mental status testing on the sideline after sport-related concussion. Journal of athletic training 36(3), 274-279.

McCrea M., Kelly J., et al., 1997. Standardized assessment of concussion in football players. Neurology 48(3), 586-588.

McCrea M., Kelly J., et al., 1998. Standardized assessment of concussion (SAC): on-site mental status evaluation of the athlete. J Head Trauma Rehabil 13(2), 27-35.

McCrory P., Zazryn T., et al., 2007. The evidence for chronic traumatic encephalopathy in boxing. Sports Med 37(6), 467-476.

McElhaney J.H., Roberts V.L., et al., 1976. Handbook of Human Tolerance, Japan Automobile Research Institute, Inc. (JARI).

Mendez M., 1995. The neuropsychiatric aspect of boxing. Int'l J Psychiatry in Medicine 25(3), 249-262.

Mertz H. and Weber D., 1982. Interpretations of the impact of a 3-year-old child dummy relative to child injury potential. In Proceedings of Ninth International Technical Conference on Experimental Safety Vehicles Kyoto, Japan.

Miele V., Bailes J., et al., 2006. Subdural hematoma in boxing: the spectrum of consequences. Neurosurg Focus 21(4).

Miele V., Carson L., et al., 2004. Acute on chronic subdural hematoma in a female boxer: a case report. Med Sci Sports Exerc. 36(11), 1852-5.

Miele V., Norwig J., et al., 2006. Sideline and ringside evaluation for brain and spinal injuries. Neurosurg Focus 21(4).

Moriarity J., Collie A., et al., 2004. A prospective controlled study of cognitive function during an amateur boxing tournament Neurology 62, 1497-1502.

Moriarity J., Collie A., et al., 2004. A prospective controlled study of cognitive function during an amateur boxing tournament. Neurology 62(9), 1497-502.

Newman J., Shewchenko N., et al., 2000. A proposed new biomechanical head injury assessment function-The maximum power index. Stapp Car Crash Journal 44, 215-247.

Ng'walali P., Muraoka N., et al., 2000. Medico-legal implications of acute subdural haematoma in boxing. Journal of Clinical Forensic Medicine 7, 153-155.

Ommaya A. and Gennarelli T., 1974. Cerebral concussion and traumatic unconsciousness. Correlation of experimental and clinical observations of blunt head injuries. Brain 97(4), 633-654.

Ommaya A. and Hirsch A., 1971. Tolerance for cerebral concussion from head impact and whiplash in primates. J Biomechanics 4, 13-21.

Padgaonkar A., Krieger K., et al., 1975. Measurement of angular acceleration of a rigid body using linear accelerometers. ASME J. Appl. Mech. 42, 552-558.

Pellman E., Lovell M., et al., 2006. Concussion in professional football: recovery of NFL and high school athletes assessed by computerized neuropsychological testing--Part 12. Neurosurgery 58(2), 263-74.

Pellman E., Viano D., et al., 2003. Concussion in professional football: reconstruction of game impacts and injuries. Neurosurgery 53(4), 799-812.

Pellman E.J., Viano D.C., et al., 2003. Concussion in professional football: Reconstruction of game impacts and injuries. Neurosurgery 53(4), 799-812.

Porter M., 2003. A 9-year controlled prospective neuropsychologic assessment of amateur boxing. Clin J Sport Med 13(6), 339-52.

Porter M. and O'Brien M., 1996. Incidence and severity of injuries resulting from amateur boxing in Ireland. J Clin Sports Med 6(2), 97-101.

Powell J. and Barber-Foss K., 1999. Traumatic brain injury in high school athletes JAMA 282(10), 958-963.

Prasad P. and Mertz H., 1985. The position of the United States Delegation to the ISO working group 6 on the use of HIC in the automotive environment. SAE Paper No. 851246.

Ravdin L., Barr W., et al., 2003. Assessment of cognitive recovery following sports related head trauma in boxers. Clin J Sport Med 13(1), 21-7.

Reid T., 2005. Female boxer dies after knockout loss. Washington Post. Washington

Roberts A., 1969. Brain damage in boxers. London, Pitman Publishing.

Roberts G., Allsop D., et al., 1990. The occult aftermath of boxing. Journal of neurology, neurosurgery, and psychiatry 53, 373-378.

Rousseau P. and Hoshizaki T., 2009. The influence of deflection and neck compliance on the impact dynamics of the Hybrid III headform. J. Sports Engineering and Technology 223, 89-97.

SAE, 1995. Instrumentation for impact test-part 1: electronic instrumentation. Society of Automotive Engineers (SAE paper no. J211/1).

Saunders R. and Harbaugh R., 1984. The second impact in catastrophic contact sports head trauma. JAMA 252, 538-539.

Schneider R., 1973. Mechanisms of injury. Head and neck injuries in football. Baltimore Williams & Williams: 77-126.

Sherman D., Bir C., et al., 2004. Correlation between punch dynamics and risk of injury. In Proceedings of Engineering of Sport 5th International Conference. Sacramento, CA.

Smith M.S., Dyson R.J., et al., 2000. Development of a boxing dynamometer and its punch force discrimination efficacy. Journal of Sports Science 18, 445-450.

Stojsih S., Boitano M., *et al.*, 2008. A prospective study of punch biomechanics and cognitive function for amateur boxers. Br J Sports Med, bjsm.2008.052845.

Stojsih S., Sherman D., *et al.*, 2010. Gender and basic boxing punch type comparisons. Detroit, Wayne State University.

Symonds C., 1962. Concussions and its sequelae. Lancet 1, 1-5.

Terrell T., Bostick R., *et al.*, 2008. APOE, APOE promotor, and Tau genotypes and risk for concussion in college athletes. Clin J Sport Med 18(1), 10-17.

Tierney R., Sitler M., *et al.*, 2005. Gender Differences in Head-Neck Segment Dynamic Stabilization during Head Acceleration. Medicine & Science in Sports & Exercise 37(2), 272-279.

Timm K., Wallach J., *et al.*, 1993. Fifteen years of amateur boxing injuries/illnesses at the United States Olympic Training Center. Journal of athletic training 28(4), 330-334.

USA Boxing, 2008. USA Boxing Rulebook. 68-69

USA Boxing, 2009. The evolution of women's boxing. Retrieved September 4, 2009, from http://usaboxing.org/content/index/1033.

Versace J., 1971. A Review of the Severity Index. Proceedings 15th Stapp Car Crash Conference SAE paper 710881, 771-796.

Walilko T.J., Viano D.C., *et al.*, 2005. Biomechanics of the head for Olympic boxer punches to the face. Br. J. Sports Med. 39, 710-719.

Warden D., Bleiberg J., *et al.*, 2001. Persistent prolongation of simple reaction time in sports concussion. Neurology 57, 524-526.

Welch M., Sitler M., *et al.*, 1986. Boxing injuries from an instructional program. The Physician and Sports Medicine 14(9), 81.

Zazryn T., McCrory P., *et al.*, 2009. Injury rates and risk factors in competitive professional boxing. Clin J Sport Med 19(1), 20-25.

Zazryn T.R., Cameron P., *et al.*, 2006. A prospective cohort study of injury in amateur and professional boxing Br. J. Sports Med., 670-674.

Zazryn T.R., Finch C.F., *et al.*, 2003. A 16 year study of injuries to professional boxers in the state of Victoria, Australia. Br. J. Sports Med. 37, 321-324.

Zhang L., Yang K., *et al.*, 2001. Comparison of brain responses between frontal and lateral impacts by finite element modeling. Journal of Neurotrauma 18(1), 21-30.

Zhang L., Yang K.H., *et al.*, 2004. A proposed injury threshold for mild traumatic brain injury. J Biomech Eng 126(2), 226-36.

Zhang L., Yang K.H., *et al.*, 2004. A proposed injury threshold for mild traumatic brain injury. Journal of Biomechanical Engineering 126, 226-36.

ABSTRACT

THE BIOMECHANICS OF AMATEUR BOXERS

by

SARAH STOJSIH

August 2010

Advisor: Cynthia Bir, Ph.D.

Major: Biomedical Engineering

Degree: Master of Science

The specific aims of this project were: 1) to determine biomechanics of commonly used boxing punches for both male and female amateur boxers; 2) to determine location, frequency, and severity of impacts for male and female boxers during a sparring session and cognitive function following exposure and; 3) to determine location, frequency, and severity of impacts for male and female boxers during a competitive bout and cognitive function following the bout. Mild to severe injuries are a known repercussion of participating in contact sports. Acute and chronic brain injuries may be a result of repetitive sub-concussive impacts. Concussions (mild traumatic brain injuries) are a concern in both professional and amateur boxing. The injury profile of this sport has been well defined however, more research is need when defining the forces exerted an opponent and how the head response to those forces. Also, female participation in this once male dominated sport is increasing and gender specific biomechanical data is needed. Maximum effort punch force data was collected using a Hybrid III dummy. Male boxers generated significantly higher punch force values for each punch, resulting in significantly higher head accelerations of the headform and injury criterion. A novel head acceleration measurement system, IBH, was found to provide a much needed method to measure head acceleration in boxers in the ring. The system was used in during sparring sessions and competitive bouts. Male and female data was collected during sparring sessions.

No significant difference was found between genders when analyzing the impacts sustained. Also, the impacts collected during competitive bouts were not significantly different from those sustained during a sparring session. The majority of the impacts, both during sparring and competition, were below thresholds suggested from published literature. The cognitive function of the athletes was collected both before and after exposures. No concussions were noted from a ringside physician's assessment; however, decreases in delayed memory and concentration were noted from additional cognitive tests administered as a part of the study. In general, more competitive data should be collected in hopes of capturing concussive events. Additionally, recruitment should focus on female participants in the future. Compared to male boxers, the population of female boxers at competitive events is sparse and the need for their participation is immense.

Autobiographical Statement

SARAH STOJSIH

PLACE OF BIRTH: Detroit, Michigan, USA

EDUCATION:

2010	MS	Biomedical Engineering	Wayne State University
2006	BS	Chemical Engineering	Wayne State University

ACADEMIC EXPERIENCE:

2009 to 2010	Rumble Fellowship	Wayne State University
2008 to 2009	Graduate Research Assistant	Wayne State University
2007 to 2008	Graduate Professional Scholarship	Wayne State University
2006 to 2007	Graduate Student Assistant	Wayne State University

SELECTED PUBLICATIONS:

Stojsih, S., Boitano, M., Bir, C. (2008) "Head Impact Accelerations in Boxing using Telemetry System." American Medical Society for Sports Medicine Conference. Las Vegas.

Stojsih, S, et al. (2008) "A prospective study of punch biomechanics and cognitive function for amateur boxers." Br J Sports Med: p. bjsm.2008.052845.

Stojsih, S., Bir, C. (2009) "Comparison of Experimental and Real-Time Data in Amateur Boxers." ASME Summer Bioengineering Conference. Lake Tahoe.

Bir, C and **Stojsih, S.** (2010). "The Biomechanics of Impact in Boxing". In: Warnick, J and Martin, W. *Advancements in the Scientific Study of Combative Sports.* New York: Nova.

CPSIA information can be obtained
at www.ICGtesting.com
Printed in the USA
LVIC04n1628250214
375131LV00017B/138